A Diabetic Doctor Looks At Diabetes: His and Yours

A Diabetic Doctor Looks at Diabetes

His and Yours

by
PETER A. LODEWICK, M.D.

RMI Corporation
Cambridge, Massachusetts

Library of Congress Catalog Card Number:
82–60832

ISBN 0-910117-00-4

Printed in the United States of America

Dedicated to my wife, Maureen

TABLE OF CONTENTS

Foreword *by Thomas M. Flood, M.D.* ix

Acknowledgments x

Autobiographical Introduction: A Doctor's Plight xi

I. What is Diabetes? 1

II. Types of Diabetes 5

III. The Natural Course of Diabetes 11

IV. Subtle Signs of Diabetes 16

V. Making the Diagnosis 22

VI. Urine Testing 26

VII. Home Blood Sugar Monitoring 34

VIII. Insulin — A Miracle Drug 42

IX. Oral Hypoglycemic Agents (Diabetes Pills) 57

X. Low and High Blood Sugar Reactions 63

XI. One of the Latest Tests — Measurement of
Glycohemoglobin 73

XII. The Diabetic Diet — Food Glorious Food 78

XIII. Food Exchange List for Diabetics 90

XIV. How to Use the Exchange Diet System 104

XV. Weight Loss 107

XVI. The Glycemic Index and the Sweet Tooth 110

XVII. The Power of Exercise 115

XVIII. Diabetes and the Woman: Pregnancy and
the Menses 123

XIX. Diabetes and the Man: The Problem of Impotence 131

XX. Complications 134

XXI. What to Do When Ill 142

XXII. Alcohol's Effects 147

XXIII. Foot Care 152

XXIV. Diabetics Can Travel! 157

XXV. Diabetes After 50 160

XXVI. Research — Quest for a Cure 162

XXVII. Recommended Readings 180

Index 182

FOREWORD

To the casual observer, *A Diabetic Doctor Looks at Diabetes: His and Yours* might be mistaken for just one more book about diabetes. This would be a serious error. In a field where instructional texts abound, Peter Lodewick now offers a superb and refreshing addition!

The first criterion for any text giving guidelines on the management of diabetes is that it be technically correct and in the mainstream of contemporary thinking. *A Diabetic Doctor Looks at Diabetes* handles this aspect well but it is the method and style which render it unique and make it a delight to read, rather than a chore.

Dr. Lodewick is able to approach his topic from the dual perspective of both patient and physician. He is not afraid to deal with the emotional issues that challenge all newly diagnosed diabetic patients and to discuss these frankly and openly. Many real people appear on the pages to follow and they give the book an added dimension. The case examples run the gamut from poignant to hilarious. Is it possible to face the challenge of managing diabetes without losing your sense of humor? The answer is an emphatic "yes." An ability not only to carry on courageously but to laugh in the face of adversity is a highly desirable gift. When this is mixed with an equal proportion of the desire to live life in the fullest sense, diabetes is not going to be any deterrent to success. As Adam Lindsay Gordon said,

> "Question not but live and labour
> Til your goal be won,
> Helping every feeble neighbor,
> Seeking help from none;
> Life is mostly froth and bubble
> Two things stand like stone:
> Kindness in another's trouble,
> Courage in our own."

Peter Lodewick has an unbeatable attitude and a real ability to laugh at adversity without ignoring the threat. This is the message which abounds on the pages of this book.

Thomas M. Flood, M.D.
Associate Director of Education
Joslin Diabetes Center
Boston, Massachusetts
March 1982

ACKNOWLEDGMENTS

I could not have written this book alone and am indebted to many people. Most important, I am indebted to my countless patients who have taught me more about diabetes than I could possibly have learned from reading a textbook. Through them, I have come to realize that although there may be such a thing as "Type I diabetes," there is *no such thing* as a "Type I diabetic," for there are as many types of diabetics as there are individuals, and treatment must vary accordingly.

I have special appreciation for Zurbrugg Memorial Hospital, where I have been fortunate enough to have my diabetes practice, and to the many nurses and other people, both professional and nonprofessional, of Zurbrugg Hospital and the surrounding South Jersey community who have been a constant source of inspiration.

I am very grateful to Charles A. Thielman, D.P.M., Consultant in Podiatry, Zurbrugg Memorial Hospital, for his help with the writing of the chapter on foot care, and Elizabeth A. Warholak, R.D., nutritionist at Zurbrugg Memorial Hospital, for her contribution towards writing the chapter on the diabetic diet.

My thanks goes to Rita Nemchik, R.N., M.S., for her constructive review of the manuscript. I am also sincerely indebted to Charles A. Suther, Director of Professional Services, Bio-Dynamics, for his major contributing efforts in the publication of this book. Through his urging, I sought the editorial help of RMI Corporation. Anne Waters of RMI reviewed the initial raw manuscript, suggested changes, and transformed my somewhat unclear wording and disjointed sentences into a smooth and readable composition. My appreciation goes also to Amy Troyansky of RMI, who enhanced the book considerably with her fine illustrations.

Finally, I owe deep thanks to my wife, Maureen, who listened intently as I harped away on points I thought should be included in the book and who reviewed the manuscript with me as my thoughts developed into print.

A Doctor's Plight

The sudden knowledge that I had diabetes was a cruel shock, similar to the jolt one feels when learning of a loved one's unexpected and untimely death. At first, such news is simply denied, but then denial gives way to sadness and a sense of loss and worthlessness. Daily activities seem futile and exhausting. And gradually, after a period of grief and idleness, the news becomes a reality which must be confronted, accepted, and integrated into one's life. If I as a doctor considered diabetes so shocking, I can imagine how frightening such news must be for a patient who has had no medical training, and who has little understanding about the course the disease can take or how to control its course.

For me, my newly discovered disease seemed astonishing for several reasons. First of all, I had learned in medical school that diabetes was a hereditary disease. There was no history of diabetes in my family; in fact, all members of my family had enjoyed extraordinarily good health. I cannot recall my parents ever being hospitalized. My four brothers (all within five years of me in age) and I had always been exceptionally healthy. We had no healing problems or incidents of recurrent illnesses, two factors known to be associated with diabetes.

Secondly, it was curious that of all the disorders I studied in medical school, the one disease I *consciously thought most about* and the one I knew I would *least like to have* was diabetes. I had learned that diabetes often underlies high blood pressure, heart disease, gout, kidney disease, gangrene, cataracts, and other visual difficulties. I certainly never wanted a disease that could be so troublesome and that could cause such prolonged suffering. I learned that some diabetics had to take insulin injections and that tremendous self-discipline and meticulous care were necessary to prevent diabetic coma or insulin shock. During this same period of time, I learned that the younger brother of one of my closest friends had diabetes and that he had to stick to a very strict diet in order to control his disease. From all this, I knew that I *definitely did not want diabetes.*

The final factor which made me so incredulous about the development of my diabetes was that in my second year of medical school I had learned that my future wife's grandmother had diabetes. Knowing the complications associated with diabetes, I was concerned about Maureen and desperately hoped that she would not become afflicted. It was ironic that *I* should be the one to develop the disease.

Diabetes is thought to be induced during periods of physical stress (such as surgery or infection) or mental anxiety. For me, it was the opposite since it was *after* my most difficult years that I developed diabetes. During medical school and internship, stress was great. It was troubling to confront very ill people for the first time, hoping to heal them with what seemed to me minimal clinical experience. This stress was compounded by the difficult, vital examinations which had to be passed in order to get my medical degree. My thoughts at these times were: "What if I should fail? What would I do? What possible work could I find?" And, of course, there were the financial worries which required me to work full time while in medical school and still be ten thousand dollars in debt by the time I completed my education. I worked long hours, sometimes without sleeping for 36 hours at a time. My eating habits were poor, and the heavy work schedule prevented me from engaging in daily exercise. Despite the physical and mental stress, however, I felt healthy, productive, and excited about my future.

Following medical school and internship, there was a period of tranquility in my life. I had finished my internship, passed my examination, decided to specialize in ophthalmology, and was assured of a residency program. Before beginning that residency, however, I planned to spend three years in the U.S. Navy as a general medical officer.

During the first few months as a general medical officer, my life was easier and calmer than it had been for years. I was fortunate to be stationed in the United States instead of being sent to the war zone. I had easy hours compared to the rigorous schedule of school and internship. I worked from 8 AM to 4:30 PM with a two-hour lunch break. During that lunch break, I resumed a regular exercise program and took up tennis enthusiastically. My responsibilities did not include caring for very sick patients; most of my patients had minor ailments related to colds or skin problems.

My family life was solid and happy. Maureen and I were expecting the birth of our second child. We were in excellent health, and our financial situation was improving. In short, my anxieties had virtually disappeared.

It was during this most tranquil period in my life that diabetes was to manifest itself. Several months after joining the Navy, I had a routine physical examination, and a laboratory technician informed me of a "trace of sugar" in my urine. I was astonished. Certain that he was mistaken, we together retested the specimen using another testing method. This second method (which, we later learned, was less sensitive than the first) gave a negative result. No sugar. The thought of potential diabetes completely vanished.

Several months later, I became seriously ill with the Asian Flu. My temperature rose to 105 degrees, and I suffered intense headache, backache, and nausea. Almost immediately, I started to drink large amounts of water and other fluids, knowing that "fluids help control the fever." And then a baffling thing happened. My fever dissipated, but I still had the urge to drink huge quantities of fluids, especially water. I had never before had such a desire and had seldom drunk more than one full glass of water per day. Even in my beer-drinking days at college, I had not mastered the "art of guzzling" and here I was guzzling, not beer, but plain, tasteless, spiritless water at an enormous rate. Along with my insatiable thirst, my urinary flow increased markedly. Instead of my usual two to three trips per day to the bathroom, I was going six to ten times per day, including several nighttime visits.

Despite these alarming symptoms and my knowledge of their association with diabetes, I was convinced the signs were psychogenic. "After all," I told myself repeatedly, "I'm healthy, I feel good, I've always been healthy. I've rarely been sick, and the same goes for the rest of my family including my parents and brothers. There is no history of diabetes in the family." I even related my symptoms to my medical colleagues so they could share the absurdity of the situation.

I continued to shrug it off for the next several weeks until some premonition made me get on the scale. My customary "skinny" weight of 162 pounds ("bones" was a common nickname) had dropped dramatically to an even skinnier 151 pounds. I decided that it was time to check my urine for sugar. Yes, sugar was present. What had been so laughable suddenly became a source of anguish and depression. In an attempt to cheer myself, I denied that I had diabetes. I ran two miles daily with the hope of lowering my blood sugar level. Not only were these attempts unsuccessful, but I developed excruciatingly painful "charley horses" in my leg muscles. (These "charley horses" frequently accompany uncontrolled diabetes.) Still, I clutched on to the denial that I had diabetes. Finally, one of my colleagues performed a glucose tolerance test on me. The values exceeded 600 mg%, the normal being less than 120 mg%. I attempted further exercise, but with no luck. The commonsense approach I used with my patients didn't seem to apply to me.

The gentle urgings of my wife, family, and friends gradually overcame my reluctance to be hospitalized. There I was, dazed that I should be in the hospital, unable to come to grips with my ill fortune. I wrongfully assumed that I would soon be incapacitated by all the ailments I had studied in my years of medical training and that I would not be able to care for my wife and children. I doubted whether I would be able to complete my term in the Navy or finish my planned ophthalmology residency.

Slowly, reality checked my bleak thoughts. How foolish could I be? "Physician, heal thyself." With encouragement from my family and friends, I decided that diabetes was not going to incapacitate me, but rather be a unique experience and lifestyle through which I could make valuable contributions.

Four years after the discovery of my diabetes, much had changed. I decided that instead of serving as a general medical officer, I would begin my residency in the Navy. During that residency, I decided to study internal medicine and diabetes rather than ophthalmology.

Much to my dismay, I was not able to continue in the Navy because of my diabetes. This disappointment was not long-lasting, however, for I was able to study internal medicine and diabetes under dedicated physicians at the Joslin Clinic who had had some 30 to 50 years of experience in the field. I also had the opportunity to supervise a large diabetic children's camp where I became convinced that diabetes did not prevent children from living full, active lives.

With my diabetes, I did not "die off soon." In fact, it has now been over ten years since I first developed the disease. Throughout that time, I have enjoyed excellent health, suffering very few common illnesses. Yes, it is possible that I will develop some of the complications that I feared so much in medical school, but even those thoughts are rare because I have a lot of living yet to do.

Yes, I have to take insulin shots. However, were it not for the discovery of insulin in 1921, my chances of survival would have been slim. I am both amazed and thankful, viewing insulin as a miracle drug which gives me strength and vigor. This attitude toward insulin injection helps me accept this minor inconvenience in my daily life — at least until diabetic research comes up with something else, which I truly think will be the case, given the tremendous advancement that has already been made.

The following chapters of this book consist of information I have gathered from my personal experience with diabetes, from my practice as a physician working with diabetic patients, and from the expertise I've observed from other physicians in the field of diabetes. I hope the reader will find my efforts helpful and, most of all, encouraging.

I

What is Diabetes?

The only defense against the world is a thorough knowledge of it.
— John Locke

THERE are over five million people with some form of diabetes in the United States. Knowledge about the disease and how it is controlled is prerequisite to proper treatment. In this world of instant communication, I would think people who most need to know about diabetes would have very easy access to helpful information. However, in my diabetes practice it constantly astonishes me how many people are totally ignorant about this disease that afflicts so many. Not only is this true for the diabetic himself, but also for his family and friends and even some of the doctors and nurses who treat him.

What is Sugar?

Surprising to many people, sugar is necessary for proper body function of *both* the diabetic and the nondiabetic. How often I hear the exclamation, "He's diabetic and he's eating sugar!" as the critical onlooker points an accusing finger. Although there is some validity to this accusation if the diabetic has very high blood sugars and poor control of his disease, it must be emphasized that the diabetic *does* need sugar just as the nondiabetic does. The problem for the diabetic is how to *maintain* as excellent control of blood sugar levels as the nondiabetic.

Sugar is the simplest form of carbohydrate and is the body's major energy source for sustaining life. Body cells need approximately 100 to 300 or more grams (or 20 to 60 teaspoons) of sugar per day.

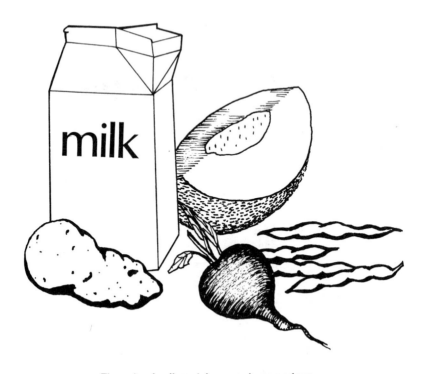

These foods all contain sugar in some form.

When we talk about blood sugar, we actually mean blood *glucose*, which is a specific form of simple sugar required by the body cells as an energy source. There are several types of sugar, all of which are forms of carbohydrate and all of which are eventually converted to glucose. These sugars include table sugar, milk sugar (lactose), fruit sugar (fructose), and the more complex sugar forms found in vegetables, breads, and starches. Glucose is also obtained from about 60% of the protein and 10% of the fat in our diet. Thus, a wide variety of foods, not just simple sugars, can raise blood sugar levels in the diabetic.

Besides being the *major* energy source for all cells, simple sugar or glucose (these words will be used interchangeably throughout this book) is thought to be the *only* energy source for brain and nerve cells. In short, without glucose, we cannot live.

When a nondiabetic consumes food, the simple and complex carbohydrates contained in the food are converted to glucose, causing a slight rise in blood glucose levels. These elevated glucose levels trigger the release of the hormone *insulin* from a gland in the abdomen called the *pancreas*. Insulin regulates the amount of glucose in the bloodstream and facilitates utilization of this glucose as an energy source by cells. When more food is consumed than is immediately necessary, excess glucose is converted to another form of sugar called *glycogen* which is stored in muscles and the liver for future energy needs. Without insulin, glucose cannot be properly utilized or stored.

In diabetes there is a deficiency or an absence of insulin production or else the body cells are unable to use the insulin properly. Thus, glucose cannot be escorted properly into body cells for energy production. The unused glucose accumulates in the blood and spills into the urine, causing excessive urination and extreme thirst due to dehydration.

Before going any further, it is important to understand that diabetes is not just a simple problem of "too much sugar." Insulin also has an effect on muscle and fat metabolism, facilitating protein and fat synthesis. Thus, when insulin is deficient or the cells are not using it properly, not only does the blood sugar build up, but if this process is unchecked (as in uncontrolled diabetes), the body breaks down fat and protein in its attempt to provide energy. This breakdown of fat and protein forms acidic toxins, resulting in acidosis or ketosis, which can be life-threatening for the diabetic (see later chapter on ketoacidosis).

The Discovery of Insulin

For many centuries, we knew very little about the cause of diabetes, although the characteristic signs and symptoms were well described. Patients were known to experience a very rapid onset of symptoms, including unquenchable thirst, excessive urination, dry skin and mouth, and massive weight loss that made them look starved. For many people, particularly children, death soon followed. Several modes of treatment were attempted to alleviate this dire chain of events, but little progress was made.

In the early part of the twentieth century, it became apparent that food and diet played a significant role in diabetes;

carbohydrates were known especially to aggravate the disease. High-fat diets were tried but did little good. In many cases, the only way to keep the diabetic alive was with a minimal amount of calories (sometimes as low as 400 calories per day) and even the use of alcohol as an energy source. Even then, the patient remained extremely ill and could barely leave the house since any form of exercise made his condition worse. This sort of lifestyle for the diabetic was indeed a dismal one.

Finally, in the 1920s, insulin was discovered through the diligent efforts of Drs. Frederick G. Banting and Charles H. Best. Thanks to their persistent investigations, insulin was found to be the substance that was deficient or absent in many diabetics, making them incapable of using glucose properly. It has since been discovered that insulin is secreted by a small group of cells in the pancreas, called the *beta cells*. Surprisingly, the beta cells comprise less than one percent of the total cells of the pancreas. The majority of the cells of the pancreas are used to help digest protein, fat, and carbohydrate in the small intestine, but it is the beta cells, with less than a total weight of one to two ounces, that provide all the insulin that is required to keep the blood glucose levels within the normal range of about 50–120 mg% (which means that there is about one teaspoonful of glucose in the blood at any given time) and allow the cells to utilize the glucose properly. It is amazing that in nondiabetics these beta cells which make up such a small part of the pancreas can continue to function so effectively despite the fact that they are continuously barraged by tremendous amounts of carbohydrate (up to 60 or more teaspoons of sugar or equivalent per day). In diabetes this delicate beta cell mechanism fails, as will be discussed in succeeding chapters.

II

Types of Diabetes

Insulin-Dependent Diabetes

AFTER the discovery of insulin by Banting and Best, it was thought that *all* types of diabetes were caused by failure of the beta cells to produce insulin. Since then, however, research has proven this to be only partially true. Probably less than 20% of diabetics have the type of diabetes where the beta cells fail to produce insulin. This type of diabetes is now called *insulin-dependent* or *Type I diabetes* because insulin by injection is needed to control the disease.

It should also be understood that even in this insulin-dependent type diabetes, there are varying *degrees* of beta cell failure. In some diabetics, *some* insulin is being produced by the beta cells, but not *enough* of it. These varying degrees of beta cell failure in different diabetics may partially account for the different amounts of insulin that insulin-dependent diabetics need for control of their disease.

Although we know that failure of the beta cells to produce insulin is responsible for insulin-dependent diabetes, it is still a mystery *why* the beta cells fail in the first place (as will be discussed in a later chapter). It is speculated that these cells may have been attacked by viruses that cause mumps, infectious mononucleosis, influenza, and rubella; by Coxsackie virus; or by beta cell antibodies that may be suddenly produced by the body for an unknown reason. Genetic and psychological factors may also affect the beta cells and make them unable to function properly. Although excessive food or sugar intake does not contribute to the development of insulin-dependent diabetes, once the disease *has* developed, it is believed that excessive food or sugar will stress the beta cell reserve, making the diabetes more difficult to control.

Non-Insulin-Dependent Diabetes

In contrast to the insulin-dependent diabetics, the majority of diabetics (possibly more than 80%) do *not* have beta cell failure. In fact, in the 1960s, Dr. Jesse Roth from the National Institute of Health made the tremendous discovery that most diabetics produce at least normal or higher than normal amounts of insulin. This may sound confusing since it would seem that if normal amounts of insulin are produced, there should be no diabetes. However, research stemming from Dr. Roth's work has shown that diabetes can still exist despite normal amounts of insulin if the insulin is not functioning effectively. For insulin to be effective, it must attach itself to the different body cells (such as muscle, liver, fat, or white blood cells) at *receptor sites*. If the receptor sites are defective or if there are not enough of them, then the body resists the effect of insulin *(insulin resistance)* and the blood glucose levels rise. Since insulin is present in this type of diabetes, insulin injections are not usually needed. This form of diabetes is now referred to as *non-insulin-dependent* or *Type II diabetes*.

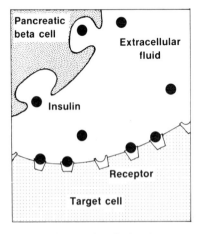

Normal insulin level.

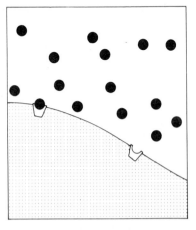

Increased insulin level due to fewer receptor sites, as in Type II diabetes.

Other Distinctions Between Insulin-Dependent and Non-Insulin-Dependent Diabetes

Another difference between the insulin-dependent and non-insulin-dependent type of diabetes relates to average age of onset. The insulin-dependent form was originally called "juvenile diabetes" since it typically occurred in people under the age of 25. In contrast, the non-insulin-dependent type was frequently referred to as "adult-onset diabetes" because of its tendency to occur in people over the age of 30.

There are important exceptions to this "adult-onset" vs "juvenile-onset" terminology, however. Insulin-dependent diabetes *can* occur in middle or late adulthood and conversely, recent studies have pointed to cases of non-insulin-dependent diabetes that have occurred in youths under the age of 20. Given these exceptions, "insulin-dependent" is *not* identical in meaning to "juvenile-onset," nor is "non-insulin-dependent" identical in meaning to "adult-onset." However, in a large percentage of cases, age of onset is often an indication of whether or not the patient will need insulin.

Another major difference between insulin-dependent and non-insulin-dependent diabetes relates to the degree of fluctuation of glucose levels. In non-insulin-dependent diabetes, the blood glucose level may run as high as 320 mg%, but it may not vary much throughout the day; it may be 320 in the morning, 330 at noon, and 300 in the evening. It seems that glucose levels are not affected greatly by daily changes of food intake or activity. In contrast, there can be marked fluctuations in blood glucose levels for some insulin-dependent diabetics despite very little variation in activity or diet. Levels can go from 50 mg% up to 600 and back to 50 all in the same day.

A final difference that I'd like to mention concerns heredity. There tends to be a much more distinct hereditary factor in the non-insulin-dependent diabetic. I have seen as many as six brothers or sisters who all have non-insulin-dependent diabetes. This hereditary pattern is much less apparent in insulin-dependent diabetes. A child may develop insulin-dependent diabetes when there is absolutely no family history of the disease. Again, there are exceptions. I have seen several families in my own practice where two or more children developed insulin-dependent diabetes under the age of ten. Thus, it is apparent that heredity, age, glucose level fluctuation, and many other factors seem to have some correlation to the type of diabetes that develops, but there are no absolute, hard and fast rules at this point in our understanding of diabetes.

Below is a summary chart which highlights the major differences between insulin-dependent and non-insulin-dependent diabetes.

INSULIN-DEPENDENT VS NON-INSULIN-DEPENDENT DIABETES

	Insulin-Dependent	Non-Insulin-Dependent
Age of Onset	Usually less than 20 years, but can be any age	Usually over 30 years, but a small number of cases develop the disease before the age of 30
"Tip-Off"	Abrupt onset of symptoms with weight loss	Slow onset of symptoms, sometimes with weight gain
Family History	At first, may be none, but as years pass, family history may manifest itself as a factor	Commonly a factor
Stability	Not very stable; must closely monitor changes in insulin, exercise, and food intake which affect blood sugar markedly	More stable; changes in insulin, exercise, and food have much less dramatic effect on blood sugar
Control of Disease	Difficult	Less difficult
Complications	May occur	May occur
Diet	Vitally important	Important, and may determine whether or not patient needs insulin or pills
Insulin Need	Yes — 100%	Needed in only 20-30% of cases
Need for Pills	No	Sometimes

Besides the differentiation between insulin-dependent and non-insulin-dependent diabetes, there are other terms that come up frequently when diabetes is discussed. These terms are discussed below.

Prediabetes

"Prediabetes" has been a term used to describe a person who is basically healthy but who will eventually develop diabetes. The problem is that there is still no way of predicting accurately who will develop diabetes. The chances are much higher in children whose parents both have diabetes, or in the identical twin of a diabetic, but even here, there is no perfect correlation. Individuals who have strong family histories of diabetes are being studied very closely in many centers around the world in an effort to pinpoint the predisposing factors of diabetes and uncover the actual cause of the disease.

Chemical Diabetes or Impaired Glucose Tolerance

"Chemical diabetes" refers to a condition in which blood glucose abnormality or "glucose intolerance" is confirmed by laboratory tests but overt diabetic symptoms are not present. There are two stages of chemical diabetes: latent and pure. In *latent chemical diabetes*, the glucose intolerance (or abnormal blood sugar) is induced by stress, pregnancy, drugs, surgery, or infection, but the glucose intolerance disappears under more normal basal conditions. Latent diabetes may progress to another stage, *pure chemical diabetes*, where blood sugar is elevated after fasting. It is most important that individuals with these forms of glucose intolerance avoid overeating, obesity, and certain medicines (unless recommended by a physician) because these forms of diabetes can progress to overt diabetes. Then again, I have seen some patients with chemical diabetes who have participated in studies for up to 50 years and who have had *none* of the complications that are normally seen in overt diabetes. Exceptions, exceptions!

Overt Diabetes

"Overt diabetes" refers to the symptomatic onset of diabetes. Many cases of overt diabetes are not known to have been preceded by glucose intolerance. These cases are often characterized by abrupt onset with frequent urination, excess hunger and thirst, and weight loss. Sometimes (especially in very young children), these symptoms may be present for only one to two days before diabetic coma develops. These cases are especially typical of insulin-dependent diabetes.

In contrast, the symptoms of adult-onset, non-insulin-dependent diabetes may be very subtle, and the patient may have diabetes for many years without knowing it. Adult-onset diabetes is usually associated with obesity, fatigue, increased urination, and excessive thirst. Some adult-onset diabetics will have a rather abrupt onset more characteristic of "juvenile diabetes," and may in fact become insulin-dependent. Anyone who has a family history of diabetes should know about the characteristic symptoms of this disease (see discussion under "Subtle Signs of Diabetes"). With this knowledge, primary or hereditary diabetes can be diagnosed and treated earlier, possibly resulting in fewer complications.

Secondary Diabetes (Glucose Intolerance Associated with Other Conditions)

Secondary diabetes is a type of diabetes which is induced by other conditions or disorders. The most obvious example is diabetes induced by surgical removal of the pancreas or by destruction of pancreatic tissue due to tumor, inflammation, or infection. In addition, there are several other disorders that affect body metabolism in such a way that diabetes can develop. These disorders include overactive thyroid gland, overactive pituitary gland (producing too much growth hormone), and overactive adrenal gland (producing too much cortisol or adrenaline). Proper treatment of these underlying endocrine disorders usually causes diabetic symptoms to disappear, unless the patient has underlying primary diabetes as well.

Other conditions which may induce diabetes include excessive or prolonged use of alcohol, malnutrition, and use of certain pills, especially birth control pills, water pills (diuretics), diet pills, and several other medications. Obviously, not all people who drink excessive alcohol or use pills will develop diabetes. The point is that those with an *underlying predisposition* may develop diabetic symptoms that often disappear with abstention from alcohol and the above-mentioned drugs.

III
The Natural Course of Diabetes

AS you will discover, the course of diabetes is a winding one, and no two cases of it will be the same. Each diabetic has a unique personality, physique, metabolism, and attitude toward diet, exercise, and life in general. Since these factors influence diabetes, the course of the disease will vary with the individual. In some respects, the diabetic must be his own doctor, for it is impossible for his physician to understand all the moods, activities, and social situations that will affect him. The more the diabetic knows about himself, about diabetes, and about the interrelationships of diet, food, exercise, moods, and blood sugar, the more able he will be to direct the course of his condition.

Factors which precipitate diabetes have not been isolated. Heredity, viruses, infections, and emotional problems have all been implicated, but the fact that onset occurs at ages ranging from six months to 68 years is still puzzling. Without an easy explanation for the onset of diabetes, the development of the disease is usually a shock to most people. Accustomed to good health, it is hard for them to believe that diabetes can suddenly present itself. Unfortunately, because some people deny that they have diabetes, they fail to learn basic information which can benefit them enormously. By learning about these complications, the diabetic may be much more motivated to learn how to avoid them.

Course of Insulin-Dependent Diabetes

Insulin-dependent diabetes usually presents itself with intense symptoms of thirst, excessive urination, dry mouth, loss of energy, fatigue, weight loss, muscle cramps, and blood sugars over 300 mg%. If diabetes is not diagnosed soon enough, these symptoms can progress to diabetic coma or ketoacidosis (see Chapter X). This form of diabetes occurs most commonly in younger people, but I have seen exceptions wherein it occurs in people in their 70s. In most cases, the symptoms are present for three months or less prior to diagnosis. Occasionally, the symptoms can be so severe that they progress to coma within 24 hours, the patient having had no apparent symptoms a day earlier.

Once the diagnosis is made, diet and insulin injections are needed, and the symptoms rapidly disappear. Diabetes may then go into what is called a "remission" or "honeymoon" phase. The more overweight the person, the more likely that remission will occur. Even children can have this phase of diabetes. During this remission phase, the pancreas secretes insulin again and the need for insulin injections decreases and may actually disappear.

During remission, patients frequently have trouble believing they do in fact have diabetes. It is not uncommon for patients or the parents of a child with diabetes to wonder whether the diagnosis might have been mistaken and, understandably, to hope that it was. For a while, their hope may seem justified as blood sugars remain near normal. However, the period of remission ends (generally within two years but occasionally after a longer period), and blood sugar again goes up, requiring increased amounts of insulin. What terminates the remission phase is as little understood as what causes diabetes to occur in the first place, but factors such as acute infections, growth of the patient, and body changes related to adolescence are thought to be influential.

Another critical factor is diet. Although diet has *nothing* to do with *causing* this type of diabetes, it has a major effect on the remission phase. Over and over again, I have seen cases in which overeating has exacerbated the underlying tendency toward diabetes and shortened the period of remission. Therefore, it is very important to plan the diet carefully, maintaining ideal weight and maximum strength without overeating or undereating.

As the remission phase ends, the diabetes becomes less stable as the pancreas secretes varying amounts of insulin. Insulin by injection may be needed in increased amounts. The diabetes may then develop into what is called "brittle diabetes," wherein blood sugar can go from 100 to 600 mg% and back to 100 all in the same day with little change in activity, insulin, or exercise.

In the course of insulin-dependent diabetes, certain associated medical problems may occur. However, it must be emphasized, *many* of them *are avoidable*. Two major conditions which can usually be prevented are diabetic coma from ketoacidosis or from hypoglycemia. These conditions will be discussed in more detail in a separate chapter, but some introductory points should be made here.

Ketoacidosis results from a lack of insulin which causes elevated blood sugars and breakdown of fat into dangerous keto-acid bodies. I have seen patients hospitalized repeatedly with this potentially fatal condition and cannot understand why they let it happen. Ketoacidosis may be caused by omission of the patient's usual insulin dose, by overeating, or by a major illness such as pneumonia or kidney infection. Often, the patient simply does not know he has diabetes and therefore does not recognize the symptoms or know how to prevent their progression to coma. In practically every case, ketoacidosis can be prevented if care is taken, as will be discussed more thoroughly in the chapter entitled "Low and High Blood Sugar Reactions."

The other type of diabetic coma, the effect of *hypoglycemia* or low blood sugar (usually less than 40 mg%), results from too much insulin, excessive exercise, or too little food. It is my experience that *most cases* of this type of coma are also completely avoidable. Most of the cases I have seen occurred in people who did not have adequate knowledge of insulin, food, exercise, and their interaction, and did not use urine testing or blood sugar testing as a guide to controlling their blood sugars. (Again, please refer to later chapter on low and high blood sugar reactions.) It is reassuring to know that most cases of hypoglycemia are mild and easily reversible, and even the more severe ones do not cause permanent damage. However, they are unpleasant and can be embarrassing.

As for the long-term complications associated with insulin-dependent diabetes, the following can occur: loss of vision due to bleeding in the eye, heart disease, neuropathy, neuritis, impotence, kidney disease, and blood vessel disease of the legs which causes increased susceptibility to infection and gangrene of the legs and feet. Cataract formation does not necessarily occur in a greater percentage of diabetics than of the general population, but it tends to occur at an earlier age. Up to 8% of insulin-dependent diabetics lose vision as a result of their disease. However, as discussed in the section on complications, potential vision loss can usually be prevented.

At present, heart disease is the primary cause of death in diabetics. Elevated blood sugars and lack of exercise, along with the high-fat diet that has been the traditional diet of the diabetic, are, in my opinion, factors that accelerate heart disease in diabetics. As discussed later in this book, diets low in cholesterol and saturated fat and high in complex carbohydrates and fiber are now recommended to prevent heart and vascular disease.

Despite the prevalence of the foregoing complications, not all insulin-dependent diabetics will develop them. Many of these diabetics have lived over 50 years without suffering any of the major complications. In fact, the Joslin Clinic in Boston, the largest center in the world for the study and treatment of diabetes, gives awards to patients who have had diabetes for over 50 years. They have given this award to hundreds of patients with diabetes. It *can* be done!

Course of Non-Insulin-Dependent Diabetes

The course of non-insulin-dependent diabetes is somewhat different from that of insulin-dependent diabetes. Since the onset is not as acute and blood sugars are not as high, the diabetic may tolerate his symptoms for a long time, thus delaying diagnosis. Because the symptoms are hard to detect (see chapter titled "Subtle Signs of Diabetes"), it is possible for years to pass before the diagnosis is made. Some of the symptoms include fatigue, which the patient may attribute to "just getting older," and weight gain, passed off as "middle-age spread." The increased thirst associated with high blood sugar becomes so constant that the patient may consider it normal, stating, "I've always been thirsty." Finally (often at the urging of a spouse), the patient has a medical checkup and the diagnosis is made. Unfortunately, when diabetes has already been present for some time, complications may also be present at diagnosis. It is not uncommon, for instance, to find indications of heart disease, vascular disease, impotence, or small blood vessel disease at the time of diagnosis.

At this point, I would like to reassure you that the diagnosis of diabetes does not mean instant defeat necessitating a total change in lifestyle. The majority of people diagnosed with diabetes will never have any of the major complications that are attributed directly to diabetes, particularly if they take the precautions recommended by their physicians with regard to diet, exercise, and preventive care. This is particularly the case with newly diagnosed diabetics who are over the age of 50.

The other good news for the non-insulin-dependent diabetic is that blood sugars can frequently be controlled with proper diet (probably the most critical factor in control), exercise, and possibly diabetic pills, so that insulin is not needed. Unlike the remission phase in insulin-dependent diabetes which tends to be temporary, permanent remissions can occur in non-insulin-dependent diabetes. Blood sugars may return to normal and stay that way — especially if good diet and exercise are maintained.

A major complication, ketoacidosis, is unlikely since it occurs with insulin deficiency, a condition not present in the majority of adult-onset, non-insulin-dependent diabetics. Also, since most adult-onset diabetics do not use insulin, hypoglycemic or low blood sugar coma is not as common, although it can occur with those who are taking diabetes pills.

IV

Subtle Signs of Diabetes

AS a physician, one question I am repeatedly asked is: "Are there any warning signs that indicate that diabetes may be present or that it will develop?" Diabetics frequently ask this question out of concern for their children or other family members. The answer to this question is that anyone with any of the typical symptoms of diabetes or insulin deficiency (such as thirst, excessive urination, weight loss), as discussed in the preceding chapters, should be checked for diabetes. In addition, there are many more subtle signs or symptoms that may indicate the presence of diabetes. Some of these signs and symptoms are discussed below.

Skin Changes

Infections or skin changes are often the initial sign of diabetes, occurring in probably over 25% of diabetics who have poor control of their disease. Boils or skin abscesses are bacterial infections that may become severe in a person with diabetes. If untreated, these boils can spread internally and have serious consequences.

Fungal infections may also point to diabetes. Again, these infections are very common in poorly controlled diabetes. If the fungal infection becomes severe enough, it may cause "breaks" in the skin which can then become infected with bacteria. *Candida* or *Monilia* fungus is one of the most common types of fungus in the diabetic because this fungus seems to thrive in a high-sugar environment. Presence of this fungus is evident by redness, itching, and malodor. Because the fungus prefers moist areas of the body, common sites of infection include the feet, vagina, and genital areas. Unless the diabetes is better controlled, these infections are difficult to treat.

Another skin lesion that signals diabetes is the "shin spot," a brown, round area about the size of a dime. Occurring particularly on the leg, it is thought that incidental bangs on the shins cause them, but this explanation has not been proven.

Other changes in the skin that may indicate diabetes include loss of hair and loss of sweat glands (so that the skin becomes dry). The skin typically becomes thickened and discolored, and sometimes the nails become thickened as well. Doctors believe that the cause of these changes is probably small blood vessel disease and/or nerve disease (neuropathy) which prevents the skin from getting adequate nourishment.

Pregnancy

Diabetes often manifests itself during pregnancy, as discussed more fully in a later chapter. As pregnancy progresses, blood sugar levels can become elevated, resulting in "pregnancy diabetes." This form of diabetes often disappears (sometimes only temporarily) following the pregnancy. Because of this tendency for pregnancy to trigger a form of diabetes, I certainly recommend that blood sugars be checked every six weeks or so during the pregnancy, especially if the woman has a family history of diabetes. Then, if the blood sugar level does get high, measures can be taken to assure more normal blood sugars and a more successful pregnancy.

Two other signs associated with pregnancy that may indicate diabetes include the birth of a heavy baby (over ten pounds) and premature delivery. It is estimated that up to 20% of the mothers who have large babies will develop diabetes. The extra weight of the baby may be caused by high blood sugar levels in the pregnant mother, which then cause increased insulin secretion by the pancreas of the fetus. Excessive insulin secretion of the fetus causes extra growth of body tissue in the baby. The reason for premature delivery is not yet fully understood.

Obesity

Although not all obese people develop diabetes, those with a genetic predisposition for the disease are taking a much bigger risk by overeating and accumulating excessive weight. Overeating and obesity cause increased insulin secretion from the pancreas, resulting in increased storage of fat in the tissues. As weight goes up, resistance to the effect of insulin eventually occurs, and diabetes ensues. This course of events represents the typical non-insulin-dependent pattern of diabetes. If the diabetes is poorly controlled for an extended time period, it is my hunch that insulin reserves can become depleted to such a degree that the non-insulin-dependent diabetic can become insulin-dependent.

Hypoglycemia

Another possible sign of diabetes, which frequently occurs in the obese person, is *hypoglycemia,* or low blood sugar (usually under 50 mg%). As discussed below, there are other conditions that can cause hypoglycemia or hypoglycemic symptoms that have nothing to do with diabetes. But when hypoglycemia *is* an early indication of diabetes, it usually occurs several hours after a meal, particularly a meal high in simple sugars. Upon eating such a meal, there is a sluggish release of insulin from the pancreas so that initial blood sugars may be high. Several hours later, however, when food has already been absorbed and assimilated, the blood sugar levels may drop below 50 mg% as blood insulin levels reach their peak. The blood sugar response to ingested food might be similar to the blood sugar levels shown in the following graph.

As you can see from this graph, low blood sugar symptoms usually occur when the blood sugar falls below 50 mg%. These symptoms may include hunger, nervousness, sweating, faintness, irritability, and even loss of consciousness (this latter symptom is rare). These symptoms are usually relieved by food, especially sugar foods, but they frequently disappear *even without eating food* since blood sugar levels tend to normalize due to the increased levels of hormones (adrenaline and glucagon) in the blood which occur in response to falling blood sugars. In fact, the increased level of hormones, especially adrenaline, may be the actual cause of some of these symptoms.

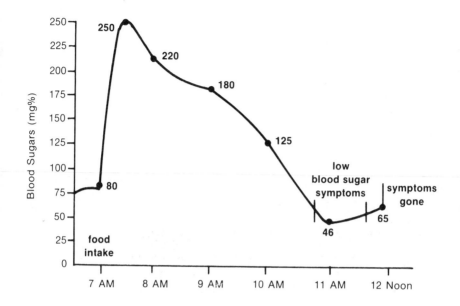

Although this type of hypoglycemia can be a sign of early diabetes, not *all* people with this type of hypoglycemia will develop diabetes. In fact, probably less than 20% will. Nevertheless, the possibility of diabetes should be explored. A well-balanced, low-sugar diet should prevent the symptoms associated with this hypoglycemia.

Causes of Hypoglycemia Not Related to Diabetes

As mentioned above, it is important to recognize that there are other causes of hypoglycemia that have nothing to do with diabetes. These causes include starvation, alcoholism, underactive adrenal or pituitary glands, liver disease (cirrhosis or hepatitis), drugs, cancer, and tumors of the beta cells (causing the cells to produce excessive insulin).

These conditions are serious and require prompt medical attention. Because of their complexity, a full discussion is beyond the scope of this book. However, the biggest point of differentiation between these disorders and those of the more benign condition of hypoglycemia of early diabetes is the *fasting blood sugar level*. If the hypoglycemia is unrelated to diabetes, the fasting blood sugar (the blood sugar taken when the person just wakes up after not having eaten for several hours) may be less than 50 mg%, even dropping to 20 or 30 mg%. The hypoglycemia associated with these low blood sugar levels suggests much more serious disorders than the hypoglycemia linked with mild diabetes.

When Hypoglycemia is Not Hypoglycemia

In my medical practice I have seen many cases in which people with symptoms of nervousness, shakes, faintness, palpitations, sweats, irritability, depression, and fatigue have been diagnosed as having hypoglycemia. Reviewing the symptoms of these individuals, however, it is apparent that the *pattern* of these symptoms is different from the symptom pattern associated with the hypoglycemia in mild diabetes or the hypoglycemia due to more serious disorders. In contrast to truly hypoglycemic patients, these people have symptoms that appear very suddenly and have little relation to food or sugar intake. They may occur in the morning before food is eaten and then last for hours or days. Upon laboratory analysis, however, these people have blood sugar levels between 50 and 100 mg% — NORMAL BLOOD SUGARS! Some people may insist that a value of 56 for blood sugar is low (for some diabetics, it *is* relatively low since they get symptomatic from this level, especially if they are used to levels above 200 mg%), but I consider this value within the normal range. It is my strong contention that it is far better to have blood sugars in the 50 to 100 mg% range than it is to have levels above 100 mg% that may indicate diabetes.

If these people do not have hypoglycemia, then what do they have? There are several conditions that can cause symptoms similar to those caused by hypoglycemia. Possible causes include an overactive thyroid gland (hyperthyroidism), heart conditions, hormonal disturbances (especially those associated with the menstrual cycle or menopause), withdrawal from alcohol and drugs, excessive caffeine intake, and some psychological disorders. Although blood testing shows that hypoglycemia is not responsible for these symptoms, many people do feel better if they omit sugar from their diet. However, it is still important to search for other possible causes for these hypoglycemic-like symptoms.

Impotence

Another symptom that may occur in the undiagnosed diabetic is impotence. Many men present this complaint to their doctor. With proper treatment, the impotence may disappear. Impotence will be discussed more thoroughly in the chapter entitled "Diabetes and the Man: The Problem of Impotence."

Vascular Disease

Finally, when vascular disease (arteriosclerosis) of the legs or heart (coronary artery disease) occurs at a relatively young age, diabetes may be the cause. This is especially true in women since vascular disease is normally very rare before menopause. Vascular disease is discussed much more thoroughly in the chapter on complications.

In summary, the above signs and symptoms frequently occur in the diabetic who has not been diagnosed. Early diagnosis can mean early treatment and prevention of some of these signs, and this is the reason behind diabetes detection drives, which can enlighten people who are unaware of these signs.

V

Making the Diagnosis

SIGNS and symptoms that should make one suspect diabetes include fatigue, increased thirst, increased urination, change in appetite (often an increase, but sometimes a decrease), weight loss, blurred vision, double vision, and other more subtle symptoms discussed elsewhere in the book as premonitory indications of diabetes. To confirm the diagnosis, the following tests are used.

Urine Sugar Test

Urine sugar tests are the least reliable of the diagnostic laboratory tests and cannot be used alone to make the diagnosis. However, these tests are useful in monitoring known cases of diabetes and in alerting patients to the possibility of diabetes if they have any of the above signs or symptoms. It is important to know, however, that urine sugar tests can be negative despite elevated blood sugar. The reverse can also be true; i.e., urine sugar tests can be positive despite normal blood sugar levels. The following case illustrates this problem.

I recently treated a five-year-old boy who was spilling sugar in his urine. The boy's family doctor had referred him to me because a routine urinalysis showed sugar in his urine despite a blood sugar of only 112 mg%. The young boy's mother was terribly concerned that her child might have diabetes. Seeing the boy, however, I was impressed by the lack of any symptoms that might indicate diabetes and by a physical examination that suggested excellent health.

Testing his urine for sugar yielded high results (1%), but a simultaneous blood sugar test result was only 71 mg%. Thirty minutes later I repeated the urine test and it still showed sugar. My conclusion (which greatly relieved his mother) was that her boy did *not* have diabetes, but, rather, a low kidney threshold for sugar, causing sugar to appear in the urine even with normal blood sugars. The medical term for this condition is *renal glycosuria*. It is a benign condition with no increased susceptibility to diabetes.

Fasting Blood Sugar Test

A fasting blood sugar is measured when a patient has not eaten or drunk anything for eight or more hours. In people under the age of 50, normal fasting blood sugar levels range from 50 to 100 mg%, depending on the method of chemical analysis. Anything above that range is strongly suggestive of diabetes, although as one gets older (see chapter entitled "Diabetes After 50") the fasting blood sugar may get somewhat higher without indicating diabetes. According to the American Diabetes Association, the diagnosis of diabetes is appropriate if two successive fasting blood sugars are over 140 mg%. Note that the fasting blood sugar can be normal or near normal in the milder forms of diabetes, but the blood sugar following eating is high. The following test is useful in these cases.

After Eating (Postprandial) Blood Sugar Test

This test will identify a greater percentage of diabetics (especially people with milder forms of diabetes) than the previously discussed fasting blood sugar test. After eating, blood sugar testing can be at one-hour, two-hour, and three-hour time intervals following ingestion of food containing 75 grams of carbohydrate. In general, a blood sugar level is considered abnormal if it exceeds 180 mg% one hour after eating, if it exceeds 140 mg% two hours after eating, or if it exceeds 110 mg% three hours after eating. The American Diabetes Association considers two or more two-hour postprandial blood sugars above 200 mg% to be diagnostic of diabetes. If the results of these postprandial blood sugars are borderline, the glucose tolerance test may be indicated.

Glucose Tolerance Test

This is by far the most sensitive test for diagnosing diabetes. It is performed early in the morning, after the patient has not eaten anything since 10 PM of the preceding evening. A fasting blood sugar is obtained and then the patient is given 75 grams of glucose. Ingestion of the glucose is then followed by half-hour, one-hour, two-hour, and three-hour blood sugar tests. In some cases, four- and five-hour blood sugar tests are also done, especially when early diabetes is suspected. The four- and five-hour blood sugar tests may be abnormally low in early diabetes, as discussed previously. The glucose tolerance tests should be preceded by three days of heavy carbohydrate intake which makes the test more accurate. Normal results of the glucose tolerance test show the fasting blood sugar below 110 mg%, the one-half-hour and the one-hour level below 160-180 mg%, the two-hour level below 140 mg%, and the three-hour level below 110 mg%. The combination of two or more results above these levels, especially if values are well above 200 mg%, is a strong indication that diabetes *may* be present. It is important to emphasize, however, that improper food intake, inactivity (such as bed rest when in a hospital), and a number of medications (diuretics, hormone pills, birth control pills, Inderal, and many others) can cause spuriously high blood sugar results. In such circumstances, the glucose tolerance test is not recommended since it could *erroneously* diagnose diabetes. Also, it is not uncommon to see suspiciously abnormal glucose tolerance results return to normal when the test is repeated several weeks later. The explanation for this is not clear but it illustrates the point that diabetes should *not* be diagnosed prematurely based on the test results alone. The overall profile of how well the patient is doing is vital to a proper diagnosis.

There is a modification of the glucose tolerance test in which sugar is given intravenously instead of orally. This test is performed only when patients cannot tolerate taking sugar by mouth because of vomiting.

Steroid Glucose Tolerance Test

The steroid glucose test is sometimes used when the glucose tolerance is normal but when there is a history suggestive of diabetes that developed during a period of stress or during pregnancy. This test may help determine whether a patient may be prone to diabetes. In the test, a steroid is given which acts like pregnancy or stress in bringing about glucose intolerance for a brief period following the ingestion of a large amount of carbohydrate. This test is seldom used by the general practicing physician but can be used by research physicians to try to identify those people who are predisposed to diabetes.

VI
Urine Testing

WITH the current trend in diabetes management of having patients monitor their own blood sugars as a more precise way of checking glucose levels, much can still be said for the value of urine testing. The majority of diabetics can get a good idea of how well their disease is being controlled from urine testing. Until the 1960s, urine tests were extremely cumbersome and time-consuming. In the past few decades, however, several excellent urine tests have become available which are simple and inexpensive and can give a relatively good measurement of the blood sugar level.

For many non-insulin-dependent diabetics, urine testing can answer questions as to whether some of their symptoms are caused by high blood sugars or by another factor, such as acute illness. Too often, patients who have not been taught the value of using these simple urine tests call me on the phone wondering whether their diabetes has gone out of control. In three out of four of these cases, urine tests would have been negative for sugar and these patients could have been reassured that their diabetes was *not* out of control.

Urine tests also save time and are less expensive than a trip to the doctor's office for a blood sugar check. If urine tests in the non-insulin-dependent diabetic are consistently negative several times a day, if the patient is feeling good, and if the blood sugar and glycohemoglobin level (an index of long-term diabetes control — see Chapter XI) are normal when the diabetic visits the doctor, then there is no need for home blood sugar testing. This is probably true for the majority of non-insulin-dependent diabetics, especially those over the age of 50.

For the insulin-dependent diabetic, urine testing can also be helpful. As will be discussed in the insulin chapter, urine tests can be used as a guide to insulin therapy. They can be used to alert the patient of potential coma or ketoacidosis when diabetes is out of control, with high levels of sugar and acetone spilling into the urine. They can also be used to indicate whether a potential hypoglycemic reaction is imminent (a negative result by a sensitive urine test) so that extra food can be taken prior to strenuous exercise. In the insulin-dependent diabetic who is young or who has a relatively low renal threshold, a negative result by a sensitive urine test means that the blood sugar is close to normal or below. Therefore, by testing every day, most diabetics can get a good idea of what the blood sugar is 365 days a year rather than the 3, 6, or 12 times a year when they visit the doctor, especially if they do not monitor their own blood sugars. In short, urine testing will cut down on unnecessary trips to the doctor for blood sugar checks. Finally, and very importantly, urine testing can provide insight into diabetic control through insulin, diet, and exercise. The following information should enable the diabetic to use urine tests properly.

The Renal Threshold

The kidneys will not allow sugar to spill into the urine until the blood sugar reaches a certain level. This level of blood sugar is called the *renal threshold* and generally averages between 150 and 200 mg%. Therefore, if a diabetic has a renal threshold of 200 mg% and gets a negative urine test, it means his blood sugar has been below his renal threshold for several minutes to several hours, depending on when he last voided. This is demonstrated in Graph #1.

If the same person has a *positive* urine sugar, it means his blood sugar has been above 200 mg% for a period of time prior to the time of voiding. As indicated in Graph #2, the patient's kidneys would be spilling sugar between 7 AM and 10 AM. However, while a positive urine test may tell the patient his blood sugar *was* high, it may not tell him if it is *still* high. In this second example, the blood sugar is less than 120 mg% at 11 AM even though his urine sugar is high when tested at this time. This is where the second voided specimen helps.

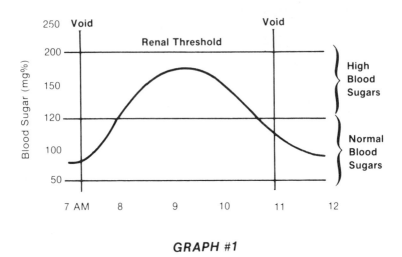

GRAPH #1

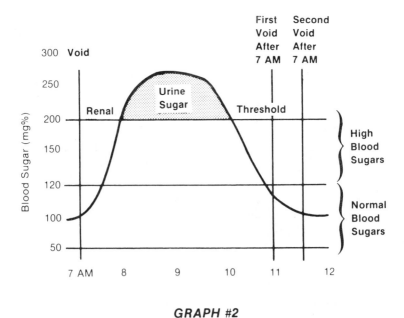

GRAPH #2

The Meaning of "Second Voided"

A second void or a freshly voided specimen may give a better reflection of what the actual blood sugar is at the time of voiding. In order to understand this, it is important to realize that urine (a product of blood filtration) is formed in the kidneys, but it is *stored* in the bladder for a period ranging from minutes to eight hours prior to voiding. Because of this period of urine storage, a *first* voided urine specimen for sugar may not give an accurate reflection of the blood sugar at the time of voiding. So, if you refer back to Graph #2, you can see how the first void contains all the urine formed by the kidneys between 7 and 11 AM, and therefore, this urine specimen has sugar in it even though the blood sugar is less than 120 mg%. (This first void technique can even yield positive results in some patients who are experiencing insulin or low blood sugar reactions.) To get a better indication of what the actual blood sugar level is at the time of voiding, it is better to discard the first void with all the stored urine and get a second void or a freshly formed urine specimen 30 minutes later. Referring to Graph #2 again, if the first void at 11 AM is discarded and a second void at 11:30 AM is obtained, it may very likely be negative for sugar, indicating that the blood sugar level is below the patient's renal threshold. If, in contrast, the blood sugar did not go below 200 mg% at 11 AM, then the urine test would still be positive.

So, for the patient who has an average renal threshold (between 150 and 200 mg%) and who has no difficulty in completely emptying his bladder, urine testing gives an adequate indication of how well the diabetes is being controlled. For these patients, urine sugar results should ideally be negative (0%). For the patient with a renal threshold lower than 150 mg% or higher than 200 mg%, urine testing may not be quite as useful, and home blood sugar testing may be preferable.

Urine Testing Methods for Sugar

On the following pages are descriptions of various urine testing procedures that are commonly used to ascertain glucose levels.

Tes-Tape

<u>Procedure</u>: Dip the end of the tape in the urine. Wait one minute. Compare the color of the tape with the color chart. If the tape indicates 1/2%, wait one more minute and compare again.

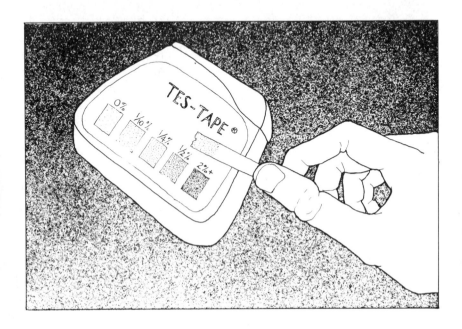

<u>Advantages</u>: *Tes-Tape* (Lilly) is very convenient and easy to carry. Since it is a very sensitive test, it is best suited for adults who do not spill much sugar. If the test is negative in a person on insulin, it means that the blood sugar is probably normal or low. If the patient is planning to exercise or be in a situation where food is not available for an extended period of time, he should probably have some food shortly after the test.

<u>Disadvantages</u>: Especially in the young or insulin-dependent diabetic, the test will always be positive, particularly for the first voided specimen. Exposure to humidity will invalidate the results.

Clinitest

<u>Procedure for the five drop method</u>: Five drops of urine are mixed with ten drops of water, and a *Clinitest Tablet* (Ames) is

added to the mixture. A chemical reaction occurs which results in the formation of a color that varies according to the amount of sugar present. The accompanying color chart shows the corresponding sugar content of the urine.

Procedure for the two drop method: This test is performed in the same way as the five drop method, except two drops are used instead of five and a different color chart is used.

Advantages: This test is the easiest to interpret because of the broad range of colors. It is especially recommended if the patient has visual problems. It is very helpful in determining whether more insulin is needed, especially when the patient is sick.

Disadvantages: The test kit is bulky. High humidity will damage the test. Many medicines such as high doses of vitamin C, aspirin, and some antibiotics will cause the test to give positive results when they should be negative since there is no sugar in the urine.

Diastix

Procedure: Dip strip in urine for two seconds. Wait 30 seconds and compare the strip with the color chart.

Advantages: *Diastix* (Ames) is sensitive and thus is similar in advantages to *Tes-Tape*.

Disadvantages: This test is also bulky. Certain medicines, such as aspirin and vitamin C, will interfere with its results, causing negative results when they should be positive.

Chemstrip uG

Procedure: Dip strip into freshly voided specimen for one second or less. Draw edge of strip along rim of container to remove excess urine. After two minutes, compare with color chart provided with strip.

Advantages: *Chemstrip uG* (Bio-Dynamics) is sensitive and, therefore, has the same advantages as *Tes-Tape*. However, *Chemstrip uG* has a broader range, reading from zero to five percent, and clinical trials have shown it to be an accurate and reliable method for determining urine sugar levels.

Disadvantages: Like the *Clinitest* and *Diastix*, this test is also fairly bulky.

When to Test and How to Choose the Best Method

When first starting to test their urine, stable diabetics, especially those not on insulin, should test before each meal and before going to bed. Any method may be used, but *Tes-Tape* is the most likely to detect sugar in the urine. If all test results are negative for several weeks, then the urine should be tested after each meal. If tests continue to be uniformly negative, then the test should be performed once per day or twice per week after different meals. REMEMBER: If tests are positive, then it is necessary to test more often. Illness necessitates more frequent testing too. People with hypoglycemia or mild diabetes with mild glucose intolerance should also use the above guidelines.

Unstable or insulin-dependent diabetics should test their urine before each meal and at bedtime. In addition, they should test the second voided specimen. For some people on insulin, especially children with a low renal threshold, the *Clinitest two drop method* is preferred. If the test gives the highest reading, it indicates a very high level of sugar and a possible need for more insulin (or less food if the patient has been overeating).

If a person is very prone to changes in blood sugar with exercise and food, he should test with a very sensitive method such as *Tes-Tape*, *Chemstrip*, or *Diastix* before exercise, long drives, etc. If the tests are negative, he should eat more than his usual diet allows.

Urine Acetone or Ketone Testing

If high blood sugar levels occur but body fats are not breaking down, there is no acute danger of ketoacidosis (see Chapter X). However, when body fat breaks down to ketone bodies, the condition becomes more serious. Tests are available to help detect whether these ketone bodies are forming. For the well-controlled diabetic who is feeling well, there is usually little need to test for urine acetone. But if any of the following conditions occur, urine should be checked for acetone:

- presence of an illness or fever;
- urines very high in sugar for three tests in a row on the same day;
- symptoms of high sugar, such as dry tongue, thirst, nausea, and excessive urination.

The procedures for three common ketone tests are as follows:

Acetest Tablet (Ames): Place a drop of urine on the tablet. After exactly 30 seconds, compare the tablet with the color chart.

Ketostix (Ames): Dip the strip in urine. Compare the strip to the chart after exactly 15 seconds.

Chemstrip K (Bio-Dynamics): Dip the strip in urine, wait 60 seconds, and compare with the color chart.

Final Suggestions on Urine Testing

It is important to *record* the results of *all* tests. An example is shown below. If you record your results consistently, you are more likely to notice any pattern that would indicate too much food or too little insulin.

	Before Breakfast	Before Lunch	Before Dinner	Bedtime
July 5	0%	1/4%	3/4%	1/2%
July 6	1/2%	1/4%	0%	0%
July 7	0%	0%	1/4%	0%
July 8	1/4%	0%	0%	0%

This written confirmation of test results helps motivate you to stay on a diet, especially if you are getting a lot of high test results. Some people think this is a nuisance, especially when they have a good idea what the result is going to be. They know it's going to be high so they don't test. If they *do* test, however, and *see* the high results, they are likely to be more careful with their diet and they can monitor insulin dosage and level of activity.

If you are on insulin and your urine test is negative before bedtime, eat a double snack. If a child has all negative results or results that show only small amounts of sugar, he may not be testing properly, particularly if the blood sugar tests are high when tested.

VII
Home Blood Sugar Monitoring

OVER 95% of the diabetics who have poor control of their diabetes at home can achieve good control of their disease in the hospital. This holds true for both insulin-dependent and non-insulin-dependent diabetics. Patients on oral antidiabetic medication who have poor control of their disease at home are often brought into the hospital thinking they need insulin, only to find their blood sugars quickly returning to normal before insulin treatment begins. For the insulin-dependent diabetic, it is not uncommon to see rapid improvement in blood sugar levels with considerable reduction in insulin dose. If control can be so seemingly easy in the hospital where activity is limited, why shouldn't it be as good at home?

The answer is complex. A stressful environment, a hectic schedule, a change in diet, extra nibbling, or an unusually active day are possible explanations for reduced control of diabetes outside the hospital. With all of these variables, how can the diabetic possibly know how his blood sugar levels are being affected?

Fortunately, tests have been devised in the last several years which enable diabetics to keep track of their own blood sugar levels at home. With this diagnostic tool, diabetics can monitor the effect of the many factors at home or at the office which influence blood sugar levels. What does a hot fudge sundae do to blood sugar? Does the blood sugar skyrocket the way the doctor says it will? Home monitoring can help the diabetic determine the effects of stress from an examination, a job interview, a family confrontation, etc. With this understanding, these effects can be anticipated in future similar circumstances.

It is not necessary for all diabetics to check their blood sugar levels at home. For diabetics who have good control of their disease, whose blood sugars are within normal ranges when they visit the doctor, or who have a milder form of glucose intolerance, urine testing is usually an adequate, convenient, and inexpensive method of determining whether or not their diabetes is staying in check. However, for patients with poor diabetes control, particularly those who cannot correlate their urine test results with their blood sugar levels for various reasons, blood sugar testing is certainly preferable.

Blood sugar testing is a much more direct and accurate reflection of blood glucose levels than is urine testing. A positive urine glucose test may mean a blood glucose level of anywhere between 100 and 800 mg%. In order to understand this, it is important to remember that urine is stored in the bladder for a period of anywhere from a few minutes to eight hours prior to excretion. Because of this period of urine storage, results of urine testing may not match results from blood testing.

For example, if the blood glucose was 400 four hours prior to voiding and 60 just before voiding, the urine glucose test would probably be positive even though the blood glucose levels are back to normal. The urine formed four hours before would have lots of glucose in it since the blood glucose was then 400. This urine, with its high glucose concentration, would then be stored in the bladder. When the blood glucose drops to 60, the urine being formed at that particular time would not have glucose in it, but since the newly formed urine is added to the bladder, which already contains the urine with the high levels of glucose in it, the overall level of glucose in the urine would be fairly high when the urine is tested, even though the blood glucose level had dropped significantly. This explains the discrepancy between a urine test high in glucose and a normal blood glucose test.

As discussed in the chapter on urine testing, a "fresh void" or "second void" might offset the discrepancy somewhat, but there may still be some variance so that a urine test will not give as accurate a reflection of the blood glucose level as the actual direct testing of the blood glucose itself. Instances when blood glucose testing may be particularly helpful are outlined below.

Pregnancy

With pregnant diabetic women, the goal of treatment is to attain as perfect control of blood sugars as possible. Anywhere between five and ten blood sugar determinations per week may be required so that appropriate adjustments can be made in treatment. Having these tests performed in a clinical laboratory so frequently would be impractical, inconvenient, and irritating. Home blood sugar testing makes it much easier for the expectant mother.

Those Prone to Severe Insulin Reactions

Some diabetics have severe insulin reactions that seem to come without warning. Patients who are prone to such sudden onset reactions should find that home monitoring of blood sugar levels can warn them of an impending reaction and allow them to take steps to prevent this reaction.

Those with High or Low Renal Threshold or with Kidney Disease

When urine testing is unreliable because of some kidney condition, blood sugar testing is preferable. As discussed in the chapter on urine testing, *renal threshold* refers to the level of blood glucose that must be attained before glucose spills into the urine. If the renal threshold is low (e.g., under 130), then the blood glucose can be normal, and yet the urine sugar may be high. On the other hand, if the renal threshold is high (e.g., over 250), the urine glucose test may be negative, yet the blood glucose may be 230 mg% or greater. Also, once glucose starts spilling in the urine, it is impossible to know whether the blood glucose is 200 or 800 mg%! For all of these reasons, anyone with urinary tract disorders or with unusual renal thresholds should use blood glucose tests.

Children Under Two

In children under two who are not yet toilet-trained, urine testing can be unreliable and inconvenient. Obtaining the urine specimen is difficult enough, and babies, not having voluntary control of their bladders, just don't give "second voids."

Illness

When ill (especially when vomiting), insulin-dependent diabetics are understandably reluctant to give an insulin dose because they fear an insulin reaction. However, omission of the insulin dose may greatly increase the possibility of ketoacidosis. Therefore, it is important to inject insulin, particularly if there is acetone in the urine. Blood sugar tests will show whether or not the blood sugar levels are getting low. In most cases, however, blood sugar levels will not decrease substantially during an illness, even if food intake is less than normal.

Those Who Refuse to Do Urine Tests

There are many diabetics who simply refuse to perform urine tests. They may feel that it's a waste of time or that they know what it is going to be anyway. I know one girl who had tested her urine enough in the past that she felt she knew when she was overeating or "drinking too many beers," at which point it became a nuisance and a waste of time to confirm what she already knew. However, her blood sugar could have been anywhere from 200 to 800 mg% with a high urine test. If she had done her own blood sugar and seen levels of 800 mg%, I think she would be much more careful with her eating and drinking habits.

Those Who Suffer a Variety of Symptoms that May Be Confused with Hypoglycemia

As discussed previously, disturbing symptoms that resemble hypoglycemic symptoms can result from various disorders including anxiety, menopause, thyroid problems, heart problems with palpitations, and decreased circulation to the brain. The ability to obtain blood sugars at home the moment the symptoms occur enables the patient to determine whether or not hypoglycemia is the cause of these symptoms.

Perfectionists

By knowing blood sugar levels at any given instant, patients who tend toward perfectionism can understand what affects their blood sugar levels and can make adjustments to maintain blood sugar levels as close to normal as possible.

Methods of Determining Blood Sugar Levels

Very easy blood sugar monitoring methods have been devised. A drop of blood and a lab stick are the basic requirements, but a machine may also be used. The drop of blood can be obtained by a finger stick. Some people cringe at the thought of having their fingers pricked, but the British have devised the *Autolet*, which makes it almost painless to obtain blood from the finger. This handy device is now marketed in the United States. Several other products such as the *Autoclix* are on the market for the same purpose. Once the blood is drawn, a drop of blood is placed on a lab stick and read by eye or with a machine.

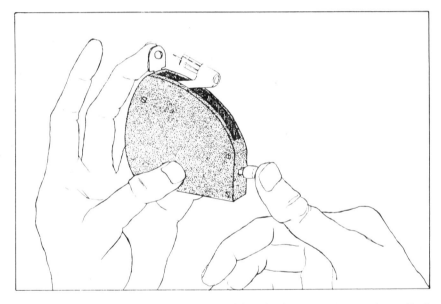

Bio-Dynamics has devised a blood glucose test strip called *Chemstrip bG*. Once a drop of blood is obtained by finger puncture, it is placed on the *Chemstrip bG* strip, and after exactly 60 seconds, the blood is wiped from the strip with a cotton swab. One minute later, two colors will appear on the strip. By comparing these colors with those on a color strip, a very good estimate of the blood sugar can be made. Most people who have been using *Chemstrip bG* have been very satisfied with both the results and the cost. The cost of each blood sugar determination is approximately 50 cents a test, compared to the $4.00 to $10.00 per test if the blood sugar is obtained in a lab or doctor's office.

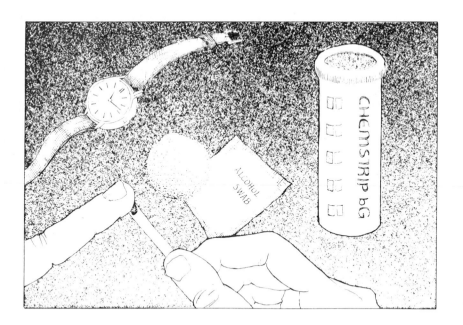

In addition to *Chemstrip bG*, Bio-Dynamics also manufactures a meter called *Accu-Chek bG*. With this meter, a very accurate determination of the blood sugar can be made since the meter reads out an exact number, such as 92, 104, or, if the diabetes is not well controlled, 212. The *Accu-Chek bG* is ideal for the diabetic perfectionists of the world!

When using the *Accu-Chek bG*, a drop of blood is obtained, placed for one minute on the *Chemstrip bG* test strip, and wiped off. The test strip is inserted one minute later into the *Accu-Chek bG* monitor, which will then give the result as a digital readout. In addition, *Accu-Chek bG* is lightweight, portable, and battery-operated and features a unique automatic calibration system.

The Ames Company also manufactures a blood glucose meter called the *Dextrometer*, which, like the *Accu-Chek bG*, is easily used. With this method, a drop of blood is placed for exactly 60 seconds on a *Dextrostix* and then washed off. The *Dextrostix* is then inserted into the *Dextrometer*, and a digital readout of the actual blood sugar appears.

The Ames Company has since made some improvements in their *Dextrometer* in the sequel to it, which is called the *Glucometer*. This device is even easier to use since it is more compact, and it is battery-operated so that it doesn't have to be warmed up prior to use. I suspect that soon there will be several other newer and less expensive devices available as patients recognize the importance of testing their own blood sugars.

In summary, home blood sugar monitoring adds a new dimension to the control of diabetes, especially in pregnant women, in children, in those with unusual renal threshold levels, and in insulin reaction-prone individuals. With home blood sugar testing, adjustment can be made in insulin dose or dietary habits to afford better control. In addition, it makes it possible for the diabetic to determine whether or not symptoms are due to low or high blood sugar. The simplicity and reasonable cost of the blood testing equipment makes home blood sugar monitoring a tremendously helpful aid to the diabetic. As stated by many diabetics who use self blood sugar testing, "I know where I'm at."

Accuracy of Home Blood Sugar Monitoring Comes to the Fore

The following case exemplifies the advantage of home blood sugar monitoring over urine testing given this patient's particular circumstances. I began treating this man several years ago when he started to have bouts of confusion, disorientation, and near blackouts that came on suddenly and were caused by hypoglycemia. These bouts threatened his job as a machine operator. He was stymied by his condition and did not know how to prevent it. He did not recognize the cause of his symptoms as hypoglycemia since his urine tests were frequently *positive* for sugar after one of these spells.

After evaluating his condition, I found that there were indications of prostatism, which meant that he could not empty his bladder completely. I also found that fasting blood sugars in the office were frequently under 50 mg% at the same time that he had high urine sugar levels. I therefore suggested that he lower his insulin dose substantially to avoid his hypoglycemic reactions. He did this for a while, but when he tested his urine and got positive results, he became concerned and, thinking this meant poor diabetic control, he invariably increased his insulin dose. This in turn led to recurrent blackout sensations. Finally, *Chemstrip bG* became available. After being instructed on its use, he saw the lack of correlation between urine sugar and blood sugar tests as indicated in the following table.

	URINE TESTS		BLOOD SUGARS (mg%)	
	Before Breakfast	Before Supper	Before Breakfast	Before Supper
20 July	2%	2%	60	100
21 July	1%	Trace	85	110
22 July	2%	2%	100	120
23 July	1%	0%	60	40
24 July	1/2%	1/2%	40	80
25 July	1/2%	1%	40	160

As you can see by the chart, his blood sugar dropped to 40 mg% while his urine tests were positive for sugar. From this correlation, it finally became obvious to him that he could not raise his insulin dose based on his urine tests without the possibility of his blood sugars falling below 40 mg%. Since he has been testing his own blood sugars, his hypoglycemic reactions have stopped, and his job is still secure!

VIII
Insulin — A Miracle Drug

U NFORTUNATELY, many diabetics view insulin injections as some sort of weapon that they should fear. This is a complete misconception. Before insulin became available, diabetes was often fatal. Today, diabetics not only survive, but with proper care they can live long, healthy lives. Insulin prevents many diabetic symptoms and contributes to muscle strength and weight gain in thin diabetics. Regarded in this light, insulin treatment should be appreciated rather than feared.

I think it is important to review the history and progress of insulin therapy since this may relieve the anxiety people have about its use. Insulin is obtained from the pancreas of cows and pigs. In its early form it contained a number of impurities. A large quantity of fluid had to be injected to get a small amount of insulin. Only one type of insulin then existed, i.e., *regular* insulin, whose maximum effect lasted only six to eight hours, and which had to be given three or four times a day. Insulin needles were large and became dull through constant use. The injections were painful and frequent, and caused ugly changes in the skin, while the impurities caused skin allergies and resistance to the drug's effect. In patients who were resistant to insulin, doses well above 100 or 200 units were sometimes needed to control blood sugar adequately.

Fortunately, much has been done over the years to make insulin easier to use. By modifying regular insulin with varying amounts of protamine and zinc, *PZI* (protamine zinc insulin) and *NPH* (neutral protamine hagedorn) insulins were developed in the 1930s and 1940s and were followed by the *lente* insulins in the 1950s. These new insulins expanded the useful time activity of insulin and allowed many patients reasonable diabetic control with just one dose per day.

Insulin became progressively less contaminated by other chemicals due to tremendous improvement in the purification process. By the 1970s, very purified insulins were available which markedly reduced allergic skin reactions and prevented the development of large, unsightly indentations at injection sites. In addition, the use of these purified insulins was found to be effective in preventing and treating insulin resistance, which was thought to be related to the contaminants found in earlier insulins. As a result, much less insulin may be required in patients who previously needed over 100 units of the less purified insulin.

More purified and concentrated insulin means that much less fluid is needed with each injection to obtain the required dose. Finally, insulin needles (especially the disposable type) have been so improved that they are now small and as painless as a mosquito bite. In the final analysis, insulin therapy today is much more convenient and much less troublesome than it used to be.

The chart on the next page classifies and describes the various types of insulin that are currently available.

For patients who need insulin for diabetic control, it is important to know how the insulin they use affects them. Without this understanding, there can be needless difficulties with control, and it is not uncommon for these patients to develop "brittle diabetes" when, in fact, the diabetes can be well controlled if the insulin is used properly. The following case illustrates my point.

A Cure of Brittle Diabetes

This case involves a surgeon who had insulin-dependent diabetes for several years. During the mornings he experienced symptoms of high blood sugar, along with excessive thirst and urination. These symptoms greatly disrupted his operating room schedule. Attempting to decrease his blood sugar levels, he continually raised his usual insulin dose. The trouble with this was

	Type	Onset of Action** (hours)	Greatest Effect** (hours)	Duration of Effect** (hours)
RAPID ACTING	Regular *Actrapid* (Novo) *Velosulin Quick* (Nordisk) *Mixtard** (Nordisk)	1/2	2-3	8
	Semilente *Semitard* (Novo)	1	4-6	12
INTERMEDIATE ACTING	NPH *Mixtard** (Nordisk) *Protaphane* (Novo)	2	8-12	12-24
	Lente *Monotard* (Novo) *Insulatard* (Nordisk) *Lentard* (Novo)	2	8-12	12-24
LONG ACTING	PZI	6	14-20	24-30
	Ultralente *Ultratard* (Novo)	6	14-20	24-30

Mixtard is a newer insulin which is a combination of 30% regular insulin and 70% NPH. Because it has already been mixed, it is especially good for those who have trouble mixing insulin themselves.
**Although most people tend to respond to the varied insulins as suggested by this chart, there are exceptions.

that the insulin he was using was PZI. As you can see in the chart showing the onset and maximum effect of the various insulins, PZI does not have its onset of action until six hours after injection. Since the surgeon took his insulin dose in the morning, it did not keep his blood sugars down in the early part of the day. His high blood sugars (over 400 mg%) interrupted his operating schedule. As he continued to raise the PZI dose to over 60 units, it finally started to take effect late in the afternoon or evening, and he often suffered severe insulin reactions at those times.

You can see how this case may resemble "brittle diabetes." However, when I suggested a combination of regular and lente insulin one-half hour before breakfast (so that it would take effect more rapidly) and a small dose of lente in the evening to keep sugars down in late evening, his blood sugars were rapidly controlled, problems in the operating room were alleviated, his severe insulin reactions disappeared, and a case of "brittle diabetes" was cured.

This case illustrates that poor control of diabetes can often be alleviated by an effort to know and understand the problem at hand. The surgeon simply did not know the onset, activity, and duration of the type of insulin he was using. He had not been instructed on the time course of the various insulins. I have seen countless cases similar to this where patients did not know the basics of insulin therapy. Once they were enlightened, they did fine!

Tips on Insulin Use

The following points highlight the most important information on insulin use.

- Review with your doctor the different types of insulin available and the type and dose of insulin that is best for you. Recently, it has been shown that better blood sugar control results when insulin is given at least *one-half hour before mealtime*, especially before breakfast for the patients on only one dose. An exception might be in the case where the patient awakens with an insulin reaction; then, part of the meal (breakfast) might be eaten first.

- Review with your doctor the difference between U-40 and U-100 insulin if you have any questions.
- Rotate the site of injection. Any site of injection should not be used more often than once every 15 days. Repeated injection in the same spot may lead to large lumps which, besides being unattractive, may cause variable absorption of insulin and seemingly inexplicable fluctuations in blood sugars.

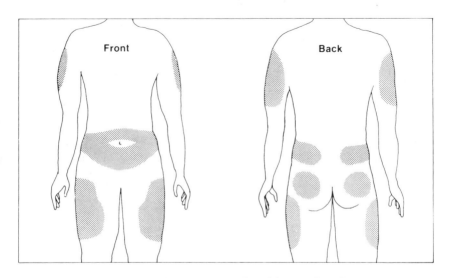

- Although the site of injection should not be the same each day, it should be understood that the insulin is absorbed more slowly in the legs than the abdomen, and more slowly in the abdomen than in the arm. Thus, erratic control may result if one day the insulin is given in the leg (resulting in higher blood sugars) and the next day the insulin is injected in the arm (resulting in lower blood sugars).
- Since no two people are alike, an identical dose of insulin in two people may have a widely different effect. *That is why it is important for each patient to monitor the effect of the insulin by urine or blood sugar testing.*
- Given the above information, it is advisable to determine how your particular insulin affects you. You should know the onset, the time of maximum effect, and the duration of effect. *You can determine how insulin affects you by doing urine or blood sugar tests that will help you determine the proper amount, type, and timing of insulin administration.*

Availability and Storage of Insulin

The following suggestions relate to the availability, storage, and care of the supplies used by insulin-dependent diabetics.

- Keep a spare bottle of insulin available in order to avoid the situation of finding yourself without insulin on a Sunday morning (when most pharmacies are closed) or while on a trip when insulin may be difficult to obtain.

- A bottle of regular insulin should always be available, even if it is not used daily. It may come in handy, especially during days of illness when blood sugar levels may run somewhat higher.

- Keep the insulin you are using at room temperature. Spare insulin should be refrigerated, but not frozen. Present-day insulin will maintain its effect for six months or more at room temperature. Room temperature insulin causes less insulin injection reactions (lumps and bumps) than refrigerated insulin (see the diagram of injection sites).

- Glass syringes may be less expensive than disposable ones, but disposable needles are sharper and less painful. Glass syringes can be used with disposable needles, thereby cutting back on the expense. It is also possible to use disposable syringes more than once. Discuss this with your doctor.

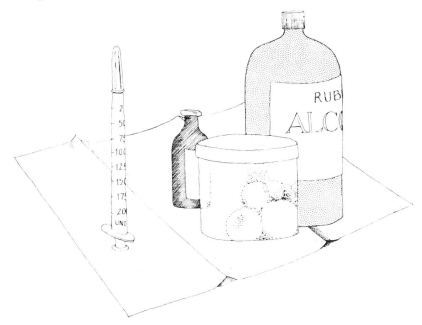

How to Give Insulin — Single Dose

1. Turn the bottle upside down and roll it between your hands. Never shake it, as this will cause bubbles which lead to faulty measurement.
2. Wipe off the top of the bottle with cotton and alcohol.
3. Pull the syringe plunger to the required number. Put the needle through the top of the bottle and push the plunger down.
4. Pull the plunger to the required number of units of insulin and remove the needle.
5. Wipe the skin with alcohol.
6. Pick up the syringe like a pencil and push the needle straight through the skin. Push the plunger down.
7. Remove the syringe and needle from the skin and wipe the site of injection with alcohol.

Mixing Insulin

Some children use a combination of insulin — lente and regular, NPH and regular, semilente and lente, etc. — to achieve good control. Whenever using regular insulin with another insulin, however, it is important to avoid introducing any long-acting (NPH or lente) insulin into the regular insulin bottle. Otherwise, erratic control will result. An example of how to mix insulin follows.

If you are on 20 units of lente and 10 units of regular insulin in the morning, and 12 units of lente and 4 units of regular before supper, you would do the following:

1. Identify both bottles and read the labels.
2. Clean the tops of both bottles.
3. Remove the cap from the needle.
4. Inject 20 units of air into the lente bottle. Remove the needle from the bottle.
5. Inject 10 units of air into the regular bottle. Invert the bottle and withdraw 10 units of regular insulin.
6. Invert the lente bottle. Carefully insert the needle into the lente bottle and withdraw the 20 units of lente. Remember, you already have 10 units of regular insulin in the syringe, so you must pull the plunger back to the 30 unit mark in order to mix the 20 units of lente with the 10 units of regular.
7. Inject the insulin.

For the pre-supper dose, you would follow the same general procedure but substitute the different numbers for the different insulin units.

Comments: If you are using relatively small amounts of regular insulin, the danger of contaminating the intermediate-acting insulin with small amounts of regular insulin when mixing the insulins is probably insignificant, but care should still be taken.

HOW TO ADJUST THE INSULIN DOSE

Some diabetics can change their own insulin dose. However, before doing so, they should check with their doctors, make sure they are not overeating, and understand the insulin or insulins they are using. To adjust insulin, the guidelines below may be helpful.

— Using Urine Tests as a Guide

Increasing Dose for Those on AM Dose Only

If, while following a proper diet, the second voided urine test before lunch is high for three days or more, regular or semilente insulin can be added or increased by 2 units.

If the second voided urine test is very high before supper for three consecutive days, lente or NPH can be increased by 2 units.

If the second voided test before breakfast is very high for three consecutive days (and the patient is suffering no insulin reactions during the day), NPH, lente, PZI, or ultralente can be increased by 2 units.

Increasing Dose for Those on AM and PM Doses

If, while following a proper diet, the second voided pre-lunch urine test is positive for three consecutive days, the AM regular or semilente can be increased by 2 units the next day.

If the pre-supper urine test is positive for three consecutive days, the AM NPH or lente can be increased by 2 units the next day.

If the bedtime urine is positive for three consecutive days, the regular or semilente insulin before supper can be increased by 2 units the next day.

If the pre-breakfast urine is positive for sugar for three consecutive days, the NPH or lente pre-supper dose can be increased by 2 units the next day.

Decreasing Dose

Insulin dose can also be decreased. A diabetic may do so under the advice of the physician. In general, if an insulin reaction occurs and the diabetic has not had more than the usual amount of exercise nor skipped any meals (these are frequently the explanations, and therefore, the diabetic need not change the insulin dose), insulin can be decreased by 2 to 4 units. The type of insulin decreased will depend on the time that the reactions occur. For instance, those diabetics on an AM dose only would decrease the regular or semilente insulin by 2 to 4 units if the reaction occurs around noon or before. They would decrease the NPH, lente, ultralente, or PZI by 2 to 4 units if the reaction occurs in the late afternoon, evening, or night.

Those who take both AM and PM doses should decrease the appropriate insulin by 2 to 4 units according to the time the reaction occurs. For instance, if it occurs before noon, regular or semilente should be decreased the next day before breakfast. If the reaction occurs after supper, but before bed, the regular or semilente should be decreased before supper the next day. And finally, if the reaction takes place late at night or before breakfast, the NPH or lente should be decreased before supper the next day.

— Using Home Blood Sugar Monitoring as a Guide

As discussed in a previous chapter, diabetes is often brought under control very rapidly in the hospital. This success usually results from the stable circumstances there — a regular, calculated diet; constant activity so that the body is burning roughly the same number of calories each day; and alleviation from outside stress. In addition, the doctor makes frequent determinations of blood sugars in order to make appropriate adjustments in insulin dose.

In the past, the doctor discharged the patient once the diabetes was brought under control, only to find that the disease proceeded to go out of control again. Today, however, the patient has the same testing devices available at home as the doctor has in the hospital. So why not monitor your own blood sugars? Once you get the okay from your doctor, you can make some changes in insulin dose based upon blood sugar results. If you are on a regular diet and not overeating, if your activities are relatively constant (for heavy exercise, you may have to eat more food or decrease your insulin dose), and if you understand the insulin or insulins you are using (see chart on insulin actions), you can adjust your own insulin. It should be understood that individual patients need different amounts and different types of insulin. We don't yet know why one 140-pound person may need just 15 units of insulin in one dose of intermediate-acting insulin like NPH, whereas another 140-pound person may need 50 units in two or more doses with a combination of regular and an intermediate insulin to achieve good control.

Increasing Dose for Those on AM Dose Only

If, while following the proper diet, the pre-lunch blood sugar is over 200 mg% for three consecutive days and the other blood sugars are good, 2 units of regular or semilente insulin can be added, or the semilente or regular insulin can be increased by 2 units (if the person is already on it) to the pre-breakfast longer-acting insulin.

Date	7 AM	11 AM	3 PM	9 PM
	Blood Sugars			
4/4	80	250*	170	110
4/5	100	240*	150	100
4/6	120	100*	180	150
4/7	90	210*	140	130

Usual Dose
30 lente in AM
*Suggested Change
add 2 regular to
30 lente in AM

Comments: The after-breakfast blood sugar is the toughest to keep under control. The body hormones, particularly cortisol, are highest in the morning and antagonize the effect of insulin. Give insulin at least one-half to one hour before breakfast.

If the pre-supper blood sugar is over 200 mg% for three consecutive days, and the fasting and other blood sugars are good, then the pre-breakfast intermediate- or long-acting insulin can be increased by 2 to 4 units. For example:

Date	7 AM	11 AM	3 PM	9 PM
	Blood Sugars			
4/4	90	140	210*	150
4/5	120	120	230*	190
4/6	130	150	100*	140
4/7	70	90	280*	160

Usual Dose
24 lente in AM
*Suggested Change
increase AM lente to
26 units

If the fasting blood sugar is consistently over 200 mg% and other daytime blood sugars are good, then the intermediate- or long-acting insulin can be increased by 2 units. For example:

Date	7 AM	11 AM	3 PM	9 PM
	Blood Sugars			
4/4	210*	150	110	90
4/5	240*	130	90	150
4/6	260*	180	70	80
4/7	210*	120	130	120

Usual Dose
4 regular, 36 NPH
in AM
*Suggested Change
make NPH 38 with
4 regular

Comments: It is possible that adding more insulin in the morning will result in insulin reactions during the day, which is to be avoided. Eating less supper, or fewer after-supper snacks, may result in lower fasting blood sugars. This might be tried, especially if there is a weight problem. If fasting blood sugars continue to be high, then a night dose of insulin taken either before supper or later at night may be needed to bring the fasting sugar down.

If the 9 PM blood sugar is persistently over 200 mg% and other blood sugars are good, then the intermediate- or long-acting insulin can be increased by 2 units. For example:

Date	7 AM	11 AM	3 PM	9 PM
	Blood Sugars			
4/4	120	140	90	210*
4/5	140	160	90	220*
4/6	90	120	130	240*
4/7	130	90	120	200*

Usual Dose

4 regular, 40 NPH in AM

*Suggested Change

4 regular, increase NPH to 42 units

Comments: Again, there is the possibility that by increasing the AM dose further, insulin reactions or low blood sugars will result before supper. When blood sugars are high after supper, it may be wise to eat less for the evening meal. However, if you are like most of us, you will seldom succeed at this, and so a pre-supper dose of regular or semilente may be indicated.

Increasing Dose for Those on AM and PM Doses

If, while following the proper diet, the pre-lunch blood sugar is over 100 mg% for three consecutive days, then AM semilente or regular can be increased by 2 units the next day.

Date	7 AM	11 AM	3 PM	9 PM
	Blood Sugars			
4/4	60	210*	90	120
4/5	70	220*	130	120
4/6	80	250*	100	100
4/7	110	210*	100	80

Usual Dose

6 regular, 12 lente in AM; 4 regular, 10 lente pre-supper

*Suggested Change

8 regular, 12 lente in AM; same pre-supper

Comments: Again, the blood sugar after breakfast is the toughest to control. The body hormones, particularly cortisol, are highest in the morning and antagonize the effect of insulin. Make sure insulin is given at least one-half to one hour before breakfast.

If the blood sugar before supper is higher than 200 mg% for two or three consecutive days, then the AM intermediate-acting insulin can be increased by 2 units. For example:

Date	7 AM	11 AM	3 PM	9 PM
	Blood Sugars			
4/4	100	140	200*	100
4/5	110	150	270*	70
4/6	130	110	230*	70
4/7	90	90	210*	60

Usual Dose

4 actrapid (pure regular), 10 monotard (pure lente) in AM; 4 actrapid, 8 monotard in PM

*Suggested Change increase AM monotard to 12 units

If the blood sugar in late evening is over 200 mg% for two to three days, then 2 units of semilente or regular can be added or increased with intermediate-acting insulin before supper. For example:

Date	7 AM	11 AM	3 PM	9 PM
	Blood Sugars			
4/4	110	70	150	210*
4/5	60	120	120	270*
4/6	85	120	90	260*
4/7	90	150	80	240*

Usual Dose

4 regular, 12 lente before breakfast; 3 regular, 6 lente before supper

*Suggested Change 5 regular, 6 lente before supper

If the fasting blood sugar is over 200 mg% for two to three days, then the intermediate-acting insulin before supper can be increased by 2 units. For example:

Date	7 AM	11 AM	3 PM	9 PM
	Blood Sugars			
4/4	290*	160	95	75
4/5	280*	150	85	145
4/6	275*	145	125	85
4/7	240*	170	130	130

Usual Dose

4 regular, 16 lente before breakfast; 3 regular, 8 lente before supper

*Suggested Change increase pre-supper lente to 10 units

Comments: It is possible that better control of the fasting blood sugar will result if the lente is given before bed rather than before supper. Also, there are occasions when insulin reactions or hypoglycemia occur after supper or bedtime. When this happens, the fasting blood sugar may get high because the body produces hormones to counteract the effect of insulin. This is called the *Somoygi effect*. In such cases, the fasting blood sugar may improve with *less* insulin. Discuss this with your doctor.

Decreasing Dose

Insulin can be decreased if insulin reactions occur. See the previous discussion under adjusting insulin using urine tests as a guide.

Diet and Insulin

Many of the suggested adjustments in insulin dose are needed when the two critical factors of diet and activity are kept constant. But what happens when diet and activity change? Here the situation becomes much more tricky. I cannot, for instance, predict exactly what is going to happen when my patients decide to splurge or consume a vastly different number of calories each day. For many patients who tend to deviate from their standard diet, I try to determine what effect the change in calories will have on their blood sugars and then attempt to make an adjustment in insulin according to the percentage of extra calories they are consuming. It may then be reasonable to take a small percentage of extra insulin to compensate for the heavy meal in order to keep the blood sugar down.

The drawback to this compensation is that if the number of calories consumed exceeds the number of calories burned by the body, there may be weight gain, especially if the overeating becomes a daily habit. Also, patients should be aware that over-eating can accelerate arteriosclerosis. Many diabetic specialists feel that the less insulin that is needed to control the blood sugars, the better. Their goal, and I tend to agree with them, is for the patient to eat just enough to maintain good nutrition and strength so that only a minimum of insulin is needed. Extra calories require extra insulin, which thwarts achievement of excellent control with as little insulin as possible.

What To Do When All Blood Sugars Are High

In certain circumstances, blood sugars can rise even if the diet and activity are relatively constant. The hormonal changes involved with pregnancy, menses, and illness can all affect blood sugar control. Since these issues have been discussed in other chapters, I will not discuss them again here. However, there are other times when the blood sugar rises for unexplained reasons. If this occurs, it is important to continue the usual doses of insulin while supplementing them with small amounts of extra regular insulin. If blood sugars are high with heavy spillage of urinary acetone, about 20% of the total usual dose of insulin can be given at frequent intervals (see chapter on ketoacidosis and sick day rules). When blood sugars are high (over 200–250 mg%) *without* urinary acetone, about 10% of the usual dose can be given several times a day until blood sugars are back to normal. Then the usual insulin dose should be reinstituted.

IX

Oral Hypoglycemic
Agents (Diabetes Pills)

ALTHOUGH there is little doubt that insulin is very effective in controlling diabetes, there is always the risk that too much insulin may cause a serious reaction due to low blood sugar. In addition, the nuisance of injecting insulin and always eating very regularly can make it particularly difficult for insulin-dependent diabetics. For these reasons, investigators have explored the possibility of an insulin substitute. Oral hypoglycemic agents (so named because they lower blood sugar levels and are taken orally), commonly called "diabetes pills," were developed with the hope that they would have the same effect as insulin without being injected. They have been used to treat some cases of diabetes since 1956 when the first of these drugs, *Orinase* (Upjohn), became available. Initially, there was tremendous enthusiasm with their use since they were found to normalize blood glucose levels in 50% or more cases of adult-onset, non-insulin-dependent diabetes.

This enthusiasm has been greatly tempered, however, by a research study called the University Group Diabetes Program (UGDP Study) that was conducted in 12 centers throughout the U.S. between 1958 and 1970. In this study, patients were divided into five groups:

Group 1: those on Orinase, 1500 mg/day
Group 2: those on constant dose of insulin
Group 3: those on varied dose of insulin, depending on blood
sugar levels

Group 4: those on placebos
Group 5: those on phenformin* or DBI, 100 mg/day

This study caused quite a stir by concluding (and announc-
ing in several U.S. papers) that the diabetes pills did more harm
than good. Because of these results, some doctors stopped
recommending these pills because of their possible link to heart
attacks. However, many other physicians proclaimed the results
of the study to be inconclusive and misleading.

One of the major criticisms was that during the course of the
study some patients continued using the diabetes pills even when
their blood sugars were not improving and they were not losing
weight, two of the prime objectives in treating adult-onset, non-
insulin-dependent diabetes. If blood sugars are not improving
despite proper diet, a change in medication is indicated. In the
UGDP Study, however, patients were kept on the same dose of
medicine (in the case of Orinase, 1500 mg or 3 tablets per day)
for *twelve years*! Thus it may have been poor control of diabetes
and improper use of medication rather than the adverse effect of
the pills themselves which could have led to the unfavorable
results. Each case of diabetes is unique; and proper supervision
and adjustment of medication are essential for sufficient control.

Another criticism was that although there were more
patients on Orinase who suffered cardiovascular mortality, many
of these patients were sicker in the first place. After much inves-
tigation, it has been found that the patients treated with Orinase
had more cardiovascular risk factors *before* the study began
than those in the other groups. For these and other reasons, the
conclusions of the UGDP Study were thought to be invalid by
several professionals. However, the controversial reverberations
of the study have had enough of an impact that most doctors feel
the diabetes pills should not be used by patients who do not
commit themselves to a restricted diet.

How the Pills Work

As indicated in the following table, there are currently four
different tablets that are used in the U.S.: *Orinase* (Upjohn),
Dymelor (Lilly), *Diabinese* (Pfizer), and *Tolinase* (Upjohn).

*This drug has since been taken off the market by the FDA because of serious
complications that can result from its use.

ORAL MEDICINES

Name	*Duration Of Effect	Typical Dose
Sulfonylureas		
Orinase (tolbutamide)	6–8 hrs.	1–3x/day
Diabinese (chlorpropamide)	24 or more hrs.	1x/day
Dymelor (acetohexamide)	12–24 hrs.	1 or 2x/day
Tolinase (tolazamide)	12–24 hrs.	1 or 2x/day

*In some patients, unaccountably very long-lasting, profound blood sugar-lowering effects have occurred.

There are other drugs used in Europe that have not yet been approved by the FDA but which may have advantages (such as greater potency and fewer side effects) over the ones that have already been approved.

There are several points to be made regarding diabetes pills:

- The pills are *not* oral insulin. Insulin cannot be given orally because it is broken down by the digestive processes before it is absorbed in the bloodstream where it can take effect.
- These pills can significantly lower blood sugar levels in non-insulin-dependent diabetics, but only to a small degree in most insulin-dependent diabetics. Therefore, these pills are currently used only in certain cases of less severe, non-insulin-dependent diabetes.
- The exact mechanism by which diabetes pills lower blood sugar is not completely known. They appear to increase production of insulin from the pancreas, but they also seem to lower resistance to the effect of insulin in many non-insulin-dependent diabetics. As mentioned before, non-insulin-dependent diabetics seem to have fewer insulin receptors. Diabetes pills probably increase the number of functioning receptors, thus allowing insulin to be more effective in lowering blood sugar.
- As indicated in the table, individual oral medications have different durations of effect. Diabinese, for instance, has an effect for over 24 hours and therefore only has to be taken once a

day, whereas Orinase has a short duration of action and may have to be taken as often as three times a day.

- Although the diabetes pills tend to be similar in structure, they are not necessarily interchangeable. One drug may simply not be effective in a given patient. In other cases, there may be adverse reactions if one oral agent is substituted for another.
- Occasionally, diabetes pills can be very long-lasting and cause blood glucose levels to drop dramatically. This effect is especially apparent when patients are sick and not eating much. Because of this possible effect, I strongly recommend that patients who take diabetes pills should not use them when they are ill unless they *know* their blood sugar level is high (by testing urine or blood sugars at home).

Who Should Use Diabetes Pills?

I have seen several cases where oral diabetic medications have been particularly effective. Especially in newly-onset diabetes where it is not certain whether the patient will be insulin-dependent, these pills may be useful in determining whether or not blood sugars will normalize. Oral agents may also be very helpful for those people whose jobs would be jeopardized if they were placed on insulin. Some companies have established guidelines wherein they will not hire or retain personnel who require insulin for diabetic control. Thank goodness the National Hockey League and baseball leagues haven't adopted such errant policies, or else Bobby Clark, Catfish Hunter, and many other gifted athletes would have been forced to give up their playing careers unnecessarily. Fortunately, there are many establishments that will hire insulin-dependent diabetics, recognizing that these people offer much talent. However, for the organizations with less reasonable policies, a diabetic's job may be at stake. I have seen several people in these latter circumstances do remarkably well controlling their blood sugars with diabetes pills instead of insulin. These people were highly motivated and knew the importance of exercise and extremely well-controlled diet.

The pills may be helpful in the older person too, especially if there is a visual disability. If adequate control is possible with the use of these oral agents, diabetic control can certainly be simplified.

Caution

It is critical that diabetics who use oral hypoglycemic agents are aware that there are interactions between these pills and other medications. Large doses of aspirin, Butazolidin (an arthritic drug), and anticoagulants (drugs which prevent clotting of blood) intensify the effects of diabetes pills. Other drugs, such as diuretics (water pills), steroids, nicotinic acid, and birth control pills, may *impair* the effect of diabetes pills. Because these curious interactions can affect diabetic control, the use of any drug should be discussed with a doctor.

Who Should Not Use Diabetes Pills?

Because many patients balk at the thought of insulin, diabetes pills are often tried with newly diagnosed patients if they can effectively control blood sugars. Only if the pills fail to obtain the desired blood sugar levels (and if other serious medical problems develop) will doctors agree to resort to insulin treatment. There are some cases, however, when these diabetes pills should not be used, especially in light of the UGDP Study. The question is: Should these pills be tried out on patients in the first place? The following case illustrates this predicament.

The case involves a man who is a 45-year-old, overweight (243-pound) lawyer who had had diabetes for about five or six years. Blood sugars were running over 250 mg% despite a maximum dose of two different kinds of diabetes pills. His doctor felt the pills were not effective and referred him to the hospital to begin insulin treatment. But lo and behold! Once in the hospital, blood sugars quickly improved as indicated in the following chart. (Note: DBI was the previously mentioned drug used for diabetes until 1978 when FDA disapproved its use.)

Why did the blood sugar level return to normal? Obviously, something was done in the hospital that the lawyer was not doing at home. As you have probably guessed, we simply put him on a diet! Stress and strain aggravate diabetes, and in the lawyer's case, this stress led to overconsumption of food. The key

Date	Blood Sugar	Diabetes Treatment
April 11	322 — Fasting 273 — 3 P M	Diabinese 500 plus DBI 100
April 12	292 — Fasting 231 — 3 P M	Diabinese 500 plus DBI
April 13	194 — Fasting 203 — 3 P M	Diabinese 500 DBI stopped!
April 14	156 — Fasting 142 — 3 P M	Diabinese 250 Dose lowered!
April 15	104 — Fasting 137 — 3 P M	None No pills!
April 16	97 — Fasting 85 — 3 P M	None
April 17	102 — Fasting	None

question, however, is whether or not the lawyer should have been placed on the pills in the first place. How should blood sugars be controlled at home if the lawyer goes off his diet? In view of the UGDP Study, the diabetes pills should probably *not* have been used in this situation. Diet, exercise, identification of stressors, and an effort to alleviate some of this stress would clearly be the most effective strategy in controlling this lawyer's diabetes, and these methods should probably have been tried in the beginning. Will the lawyer be able to maintain this healthier lifestyle? Only he can make the decision.

X

Low and High Blood Sugar Reactions

IN the diabetic, low blood sugar reaction (or hypoglycemia) and high blood sugar reaction (with ketoacidosis) can be serious conditions. But by understanding how food, exercise, insulin, and diabetes pills affect blood sugar, and by knowing how to balance these factors against one another, the diabetic can prevent these reactions.

Hypoglycemia

A diabetic usually experiences hypoglycemia when the blood sugar goes below 50 mg%. A low blood sugar reaction can be caused by too much insulin, too many diabetes pills, too much exercise, or most commonly, too little food. This last condition usually occurs when the diabetic skips some or all of a meal even though he takes his insulin or diabetes pills.

One of the most striking features of a low blood sugar reaction is the speed with which it comes on. The diabetic is feeling fine when all of a sudden he gets shaky, nervous, sweaty, irritable, and hungry. Sometimes he may cry, become angry, sleepy, confused, or complain of blurred vision or headache. If he isn't treated at this point, he may later develop other symptoms such as delirium or increased confusion; he may even lose consciousness or have a seizure.

Any of the above symptoms occurring alone may not cause danger to most diabetics and should disappear once blood sugar is back to normal. However, if these reactions occur in certain situations, they can be very dangerous or, if not dangerous, very embarrassing. If the diabetic is driving a car, trying to score two points in an important basketball game, attempting to make a favorable impression on a date or at an important business meeting, a low blood sugar reaction would be especially embarrassing.

For the most part, the diabetic can learn to prevent these reactions. He should know as much as possible about his responses to food, exercise, and whatever insulins or diabetes pills he uses. It is also important for him to realize that it takes less than one teaspoon of sugar to go from a normal to a low blood sugar level. Since a fruit exchange or a bread exchange equals two to three teaspoons of sugar, it is easy to see how skipping either exchange may result in a low sugar reaction. Also, exercise causes the body to burn approximately two to five or more teaspoons of sugar per hour. Therefore, if the diabetic plans heavy activity or exercise, he should have extra food available, preferably the quick-acting kind, like cookies, Coke, orange juice, sherbet, cake, and so on. He should be able to judge the amount of sugar contained in a given portion of food and to compensate for any anticipated exercise.

The diabetic will easily be able to learn how much he needs by trial and error. Urine testing or blood sugar testing will be very helpful in this regard. If urine is negative for sugar before exercise or the blood sugar is below 100 mg%, the diabetic should eat at least the amount of food equal to two to five teaspoons of sugar before rigorous exercise and maybe every half-hour to hour afterwards.

As previously mentioned, the diabetic should know as much as he can about the insulins or diabetes pills he is using. Most often, regular or semilente insulins have their greatest effect within four hours; NPH and lente have their greatest effect within 10 hours; and ultralente and PZI have their greatest effect 16 hours later. At these times of greatest insulin effect, low blood sugar is most likely. But a low sugar reaction can occur at any time, especially if a meal or part of a meal is skipped. Diabetes pills such as Diabinese, Dymelor, Tolinase, or Orinase can also lower the blood sugar significantly. Thus, a diabetic taking any of these pills should be especially careful not skip meals, especially with exercise.

Finally, if a low sugar reaction does occur, sugar is needed immediately. If the diabetic is conscious, he can take four ounces of orange juice or Coke, two lumps of sugar, two teaspoons of Coke syrup, or seven or eight Life-Savers or Charms. If these sugar sources do not alleviate the low sugar symptoms within a few minutes, ingestion of the same amount of sugar can be repeated. If the diabetic is not cooperative or is unconscious, he can be given a concentrated sugar by mouth, such as Instant Glucose, Reactose Paste, or "Cake Mate" (a decorative icing found in supermarkets).

If none of these alternatives works, glucagon, an injection that raises blood sugar, should be administered by a friend, a family member, doctor, or anyone else who is present and understands the procedure.

Like insulin, glucagon is a hormone produced in the pancreas. Whereas insulin is produced in the beta cells of the pancreas, glucagon is produced in the alpha cells (which are adjacent to the beta cells). While insulin *lowers* blood sugar, glucagon *raises* blood sugar. Like insulin, glucagon can be extracted from the pancreas in a powder form, available for diabetics in case of severe insulin reactions. It can be administered as follows:

1. Withdraw all the diluting fluid from bottle #1 (any syringe may be used).
2. Inject all the fluid into bottle #2 (powder).
3. To mix, rotate bottle in hands. When mixed, it will look like "sugar water."
4. Withdraw one-fourth to one full syringe of the mixture (the exact amount is not as critical as it is in the case of insulin).
5. Select an injection site in the upper arm.
6. Inject the entire amount in the syringe just as you would with insulin.

Within five to ten minutes, the person should awake and be able to eat. Glucagon raises the blood sugar quickly, but does not maintain it for more than a short period. Once the diabetic responds, he should be given food, preferably simple sugar. In all such severe cases, the doctor should be notified immediately or the diabetic should be brought to the hospital, unless those who administer the glucagon are very familiar with treating such insulin reactions.

After such a severe reaction, the diabetic generally feels "washed out," with a headache and nausea for several hours, but suffers no serious consequences. It should again be emphasized that there is usually an explanation for such severe reactions: omission of food, extra activity not compensated for by extra food, or improper insulin dose. With proper attention and care, these reactions should be avoidable.

The Doctor Suffers Hypoglycemia

Like many of my fellow diabetics, I too suffer hypoglycemic spells from time to time. One of these episodes occurred one night after a long day's work and a rigorous tennis match. I had apparently underestimated the number of calories I had burned that day and woke up at 2 or 3 A M in a sweat, feeling somewhat weak. Not feeling quite awake, I stirred my wife from what had been a peaceful night's sleep to request that she get me something to alleviate my low blood sugar. Half awake herself, she replied, "What do you want, some orange juice?" More awake by now, I replied, " No, but can you make me a roast beef sandwich?" Maureen's predictable response to that request was, "If you're alert enough to want a roast beef sandwich, you can go make it yourself!" Too tired for that, I settled for some orange juice.

Ketoacidosis

The other reaction that concerns the diabetic is a high blood sugar reaction with acidosis, called *diabetic ketoacidosis*. This condition is extremely serious since once it occurs, it is estimated that five to fifteen percent of patients will die, especially if good medical care is not readily available. It must be emphasized, however, that this condition *is avoidable* under almost all circumstances.

I have seen patients who have been hospitalized four to five times per year with ketoacidosis. One patient was hospitalized 20 times in one year. After coming under my care, he finally learned how to prevent it and no subsequent hospitalization was needed. I would like to think of myself as the hero who overcame this problem which nobody else could apparently do before, but all I did was give him some basic information (far from a heroic task) and motivated him to be more attentive to his diabetes. Some of this basic information follows.

First of all, this condition results from insulin deficiency. Most non-insulin-dependent diabetics don't have to worry about ketoacidosis since they usually have high levels of blood insulin. However, some patients who were initially diagnosed as being non-insulin-dependent may eventually develop insulin-dependent diabetes, especially if a serious illness occurs. Therefore, it is important for both non-insulin-dependent and insulin-dependent diabetics to be aware of the basic facts concerning ketoacidosis.

When insulin deficiency occurs, a chain of events follows. Without insulin, the blood sugar cannot be escorted across cell membranes and utilized or stored properly. Thus, blood sugar goes up. Elevation in blood sugar is accentuated by a process called *gluconeogenesis*, which means new formation of glucose. This process occurs in the liver when insulin is deficient. During gluconeogenesis, glucose is formed from certain amino acids and glycerol. This point is very important since it explains why the blood sugar can get high even when the diabetic is not eating any food or sugar. It is also the reason why the insulin-dependent diabetic should probably not omit an insulin dose even if there is nausea or vomiting.

As the blood sugar gets higher, the kidney is unable to absorb all the glucose and thus spills glucose into the urine. High glucose levels in the urine result in removal of water from the bloodstream. Increased urination occurs and the body becomes *dehydrated*, thus causing the diabetic to become thirsty. If caloric fluids such as orange juice (even the unsweetened kind) or milk are consumed to quench the thirst, the condition can become even worse, causing further elevation of blood sugar and further urination so that thirst and dehydration become even greater.

Other symptoms associated with insulin deficiency and/or high blood sugar include blurred vision, muscle weakness, fatigue, lethargy, irritability, and interrupted sleep associated with excessive urination. Through the kidney, there is also loss of body minerals, such as sodium, potassium, phosphorus, and possibly calcium.

The above discussion explains the blood sugar elevation and some of the symptoms of insulin deficiency, but these conditions can all be present without *acidosis*. Over a prolonged period of time, high blood sugar may add to the *chronic* complications of diabetes but there is no *acute* danger.

It is only when high blood sugar is associated with acidosis that a very threatening condition arises. A diabetic becomes prone to acidosis when a more severe insulin deficiency occurs in combination with excessive production of glucagon. Fatty tissue then releases fatty acids which, by themselves, may not be dangerous. However, when these fatty acids are converted in the liver to ketone bodies, called *acetoacetate* and *beta-hydroxybutyrate*, they become dangerous since excess ketones cause the blood pH to drop below the normal range of 7.35 to 7.44. The resulting acidosis, along with high blood sugar, dehydration, and mineral deficiency, affects cellular function. If this condition is severe enough, it can lead to death.

Because of the seriousness of this condition, it is important to understand why it occurs and to prevent it from happening. In my experience, it is most likely to occur in the following circumstances:

- In the person who omits his insulin dose.
- In the person who has newly-onset diabetes and is not aware that his body lacks insulin.
- In the insulin-dependent diabetic who overeats or overdrinks, especially highly caloric drinks such as milk, juice, or soda, so that he becomes relatively insulin-deficient even though he is taking insulin.
- In the insulin-dependent diabetic who is ill. Even a minor illness can apparently increase the demand for insulin so that more is needed to overcome the insulin resistance that develops with an illness.
- Under severe emotional stress. This is particularly common in teenagers when puberty and the struggle for self-sufficiency can cause hormonal changes that can make them relatively insulin-deficient and therefore more susceptible to ketoacidosis.
- Although I have not actually seen this, it is reported that heavy exercise in patients with poorly controlled diabetes can actually aggravate the diabetic state rather than improve it.

Knowing that acidosis is more likely to occur in the above circumstances, the next step to prevention is to be on the lookout for signs that diabetes may be getting out of control. Unlike a low blood sugar reaction which can occur very rapidly, there are many signs and symptoms that last hours, days, and even weeks to forewarn the diabetic of ketoacidosis. As discussed, these symptoms include increased urination, thirst, fatigue, lethargy, blurred vision, and irritability. As the condition progresses, the urine tests become high in sugar and acetone (or ketones) and nausea, vomiting, and weight loss ensue. Finally, deep breathing (called Kussmaul Breathing), dry tongue and mouth (indicating dehydration), and progressive mental symptoms, possibly leading to unconsciousness, indicate that acidosis may already be present in varying degrees and immediate contact with a physician is advisable.

The next step towards prevention of ketoacidosis is to give more frequent doses of insulin whenever early signs of uncontrolled diabetes are combined with high urine sugar (or high blood sugars) and urine acetone. This is a crucial step. When treating ketoacidosis in the hospital, doctors have found that the amount of insulin required is far less than we used to think necessary to treat the condition. Doctors now treat ketoacidosis with relatively small doses of insulin but the doses are *frequently* given (with very high success). The important point is that if it takes far less insulin than we used to think to treat the keto-acidosis *once* it has occurred, then it should take even less *extra* insulin to *prevent* it from happening.

In my experience, *frequent* small doses of extra regular insulin can be given if there is high urine sugar associated with high urine *acetone*. There are many diabetics who are extremely sensitive to regular insulin when their control of the diabetes is good, so that they may have a severe insulin reaction with regular insulin. However, when their diabetes is out of control and acetone or ketones are present in the urine, there is "insulin resistance" so that extra regular insulin is vital to overcome the poorly controlled diabetes. In general, the amount of *extra* regular insulin that can be given (at a frequency of every 2 to 4 hours) is 20% of the usual daily dose as long as the urine stays high for sugar and acetone. For examples:

Person A, whose usual total insulin dose is 20 units per day, would give an extra 4 units regular (20% or 1/5 of 20) every 2 to 4 hours until the urine sugar goes under 1%, as shown in the table below.

Time	Urine Test		Extra Regular Needed	Usual Insulin Dose	
	Sugar	Acetone			
7 AM	2%	high	4 units	4 regular	7 AM
10 AM	2%	high	4 units	8 lente	
12 noon	1%	high	4 units	4 regular	6 PM
3 PM	1/4%	moderate	none	4 lente	

Person B, whose usual total insulin dose is 60 units per day, would give 12 units extra regular (20% or 1/5 of 60) every 2 to 4 hours until the urine sugar goes under 1%, as shown in the following table.

Time	Urine Test		Extra Regular Needed	Usual Insulin Dose	
	Sugar	Acetone			
6 AM	2%	high	12 units	10 regular	AM
8 AM	2%	high	12 units	20 lente	
10 AM	2%	high	12 units	10 regular	PM
12 noon	0	moderate	none	20 lente	

When taking extra insulin, the following points are important:

- Once the urine tests show low sugar levels, the *extra insulin* should be stopped.
- If there is any concern about giving extra insulin for fear it may cause an insulin reaction, *home blood sugar monitoring* is a helpful guide. If blood sugars are above 250 mg%, the extra insulin is probably needed.
- The patient should *continue* to take the *usual doses* of insulin along with the extra insulin.
- The high urine acetone may persist for several hours after the blood and urine sugars go down since it takes several hours for the body to get rid of the extra acetone. As long as the

urine and blood sugars are good, there is no cause for alarm even if the acetone does persist for several hours.

- Generally, vomiting from a viral illness does not last longer than 4 hours. If vomiting should persist more than 4 hours, a physician should be contacted.

For further information, see the chapter entitled "What To Do When Ill." A diet similar to the one in that chapter should be followed until the blood sugars are well controlled.

A summary chart which highlights the major differences between low and high blood sugar levels follows.

	Too Low	Too High
Cause	Too much insulin or exercise and not enough food	Omission of insulin dose or too little insulin; infection, illness, stress
Preceding Warning	Peculiar behavior of sudden onset in healthy person, or no warning	Tiredness, thirst, frequent urination, · fever; illness frequently present
Onset	After short period of peculiar behavior or possibly no warning, sudden loss of consciousness, and convulsions	Several hours to days of above symptoms leading to greater drowsiness and eventual unconsciousness
Appearance	Looks like person is sleeping; sometimes there is muscle twitching and sweating	Person looks very sick; has dry coated tongue; sometimes skin is red and dry
Breathing Pattern	Normal	Heavy, deep
Urine Sugar	Usually negative with no acetone	High sugar and acetone results
Response to Glucose or Glucagon	Rapid — within minutes	None
What to Do	Give sugar or glucagon and call physician	Give insulin and call physician immediately

Importance of Identification

Because high or low blood sugar levels can cause abnormal mental symptoms or unconsciousness, the diabetic should wear some form of identification. This identification should give the diabetic's name, address, phone number, doctor's name, and type and dose of insulin or other medication so that proper care can be provided in an emergency. Identification forms, bracelets, etc. are available from the American Diabetes Association, the Medic Alert Foundation, and some of the pharmaceutical firms, and are especially useful for those diabetics who are prone to insulin reactions.

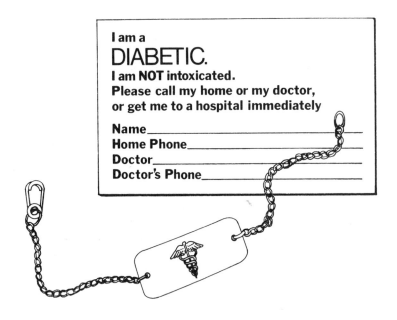

I am a
DIABETIC.
I am NOT intoxicated.
Please call my home or my doctor,
or get me to a hospital immediately

Name_____
Home Phone_____
Doctor_____
Doctor's Phone_____

XI

One of the Latest Tests — Measurement of Glycohemoglobin

MEASUREMENT of glycohemoglobin is a new test which indicates how well diabetes is controlled over a two- to three-month period. Although I originally thought that this test might be helpful strictly from a research point of view in correlating degree of diabetic control to incidence of complications, I now find this test to be much more practical than just a research tool. It can be used as a diagnostic, motivative, and therapeutic tool as well. For the patient, this means increased confidence and better medical care, as I will discuss in this chapter.

Glycohemoglobin is a substance that is formed when sugar in the blood binds to the hemoglobin from red blood cells. Hemoglobin is a protein compound found within red blood cells. These red blood cells have a life span of about two to three months. Hemoglobin delivers oxygen to body tissues and removes carbon dioxide. While hemoglobin carries out these functions, blood sugars unite with hemoglobin, forming glycohemoglobin.

Consequently, blood sugar concentration determines glycohemoglobin concentration. Also, since hemoglobin exists inside the red blood cells, and since red blood cells live two to three months or more, the concentration of glycohemoglobin can indicate what the blood sugar has been averaging over a two- to three-month period. Hemoglobin contained in one- to five-day-old red blood cells may have very little glucose attached to it, whereas hemoglobin contained in two- to three-month-old red blood cells may have many glucose molecules attached to it, especially if the blood glucose levels have been averaging very high. The different ranges for the glycohemoglobin are shown in the following table.

GLYCOHEMOGLOBIN VALUES*

Normal	4 — 8.2 percent

Fair
  Diabetes
    Control
	8.2 — 9.2 percent

Poor
  Diabetes
    Control
	9.2 — 18 percent

*as per Metpath Laboratories

The above discussion sounds scientific enough, but what about the practical aspect? As I mentioned, the glycohemoglobin test can be used as a multipurpose tool. To explain its use as a diagnostic tool, I offer the following case history.

Diagnostic Dilemma Solved by Glycohemoglobin

This case involves a woman in her fifties who had a history of good health, but who suddenly developed an infectious illness with high temperature. She recovered from her infectious illness but then had a sudden onset of severe blurred vision, making her secretarial job impossible. Quite alarmed, she immediately sought the attention of her eye doctor (ophthalmologist) who reassured her that her eyes were fine except for some refractory changes. He suggested that diabetes might be causing the vision difficulty. Knowing that there was a history of diabetes in her family, she thought this a likely answer. She tested her urine for sugar and sure enough, it was positive. When a blood sugar was obtained, results read 192 mg%, and she called me to make an appointment as soon as possible.

Unfortunately, my office schedule was filled so that she could not see me until several weeks later. By the time she saw me, several things had happened. She had reduced the sweets and sugar in her diet, her visual difficulties had disappeared, and her blood sugar was normal — 104 mg%! With a 104 blood sugar, I couldn't very well make a diagnosis of diabetes, but I was not sure what to make of her previous blood sugar of 192 mg%. Although a value of 192 mg% is high, it is not usually high enough to cause such severe blurred vision. Generally, blood sugars should be running 200-300 mg% or more for an extended period of time before vision is affected.

To help solve this dilemma, I tested the glycohemoglobin level of this woman and sure enough, it was 9.2%, indicating that this woman *did* in fact have very high blood sugars and that she had had them for at least a several week period. Although it may not initially seem encouraging for this woman to learn that her vision troubles were due to elevated blood sugars, this knowledge did solve the mystery of her vision disturbance and she now knew what to guard against. Secondly, in the weeks preceding her visit to me, she had already proved that she could manage her diabetes by dietary control. Thirdly, she could be reassured that diabetes would cause her few complications in the future, since her type of diabetes is generally mild, and when the onset occurs in someone over the age of 50, the disease does not cause many of the major diabetic complications if good control is maintained.

Glycohemoglobin as a Motivative or Therapeutic Tool

Glycohemoglobin testing in conjunction with blood sugar testing can be a very useful tool in deciding whether or not changes in diabetic treatment are needed. Many patients come to the doctor's office maintaining that they have stuck to their diet and have been active, and indeed, their blood sugar results at the office are within acceptable range. Thus, the doctor encourages the patients to "keep up the good work."

However, it is very possible that blood sugar levels can be normal at an office visit but very abnormal later the same day. Patients often have a difficult time maintaining their diet day in and day out. The doctor knows the blood sugars are likely to get high between visits, but when a patient has acceptable blood sugars at the office, the doctor has a hard time convincing him that he ought to be more careful. This is where the glycohemoglobin test is handy. If the glycohemoglobin test result is high, then the doctor has proof that the patient could do better in maintaining good blood sugar levels. I have seen patients with glycohemoglobin levels as high as 11 to 15 percent who have consistently normal blood sugars on their three to four office checks per year. If the patient can have a normal blood sugar on an office visit, he should be able to normalize his glycohemoglobin levels. By monitoring urine sugars and/or blood sugars at home, the patient can make adjustments in diet, activity, or antidiabetic agents. In my experience, well-motivated patients such as pregnant women (who know the outcome of pregnancy depends on good control) and patients who want to minimize diabetic complications *can* and *do* normalize their glycohemoglobin levels.

In addition, this test can be used to determine whether or not patients need insulin. Although some doctors believe that all cases of diabetes can be categorized as insulin-dependent or non-insulin-dependent, it is not always that clear-cut. Some patients may benefit from insulin treatment but are not necessarily prone to ketoacidosis. If a diabetic is losing weight, is weak and fatigued despite proper diet, and has high glycohemoglobin levels, there is a good chance that insulin could be very beneficial.

Finally, glycohemoglobin testing can evaluate diabetic control as good, fair, or poor. This distinction was previously impossible. With this diagnostic tool, correlations can be made between good diabetic control and degree of complications. I firmly believe that good control will correlate very highly with very few diabetic complications.

The Doctor Gets a Bad Result

After reading this chapter, you may be curious to know what *my* glycohemoglobin levels are since I have spent so much time proclaiming the value of glycohemoglobin testing. Reluctantly, I must admit that my initial glycohemoglobin result was somewhat disappointing — 9.4%. After receiving this result, my competitive nature sprung into action. Not wanting to be outdone by many of my fellow insulin-dependent patients who keep their sugar levels in the normal range, I did some serious thinking.

Although I test my urine regularly with *Tes-Tape,* I realized I had not regarded the positive results (which constituted 25–50% of my tests) as being very significant. Thinking my renal threshold was low and that *Tes-Tape* was extremely sensitive, I thought my blood sugars were relatively good even though I was getting positive results. Once I got my 9.4% glycohemoglobin result, however, I started testing my blood sugars more frequently at home.

Again, I must reluctantly admit that I was frequently getting test results of blood sugar levels between 200 and 320 mg%, especially after breakfast. I explored this problem as I would with my patients and came to the conclusion that I was simply overeating. By cutting out the extra snacking and some of the extra portions, my blood sugars dropped towards normal — the same result my patients experience when they stop overeating. Not only that, but my glycohemoglobin dropped to *6.1%* and I succeeded in rivaling some of my better controlled diabetic patients!

XII

The Diabetic Diet —
Food Glorious Food

THERE is a lot of talk about food in relation to diabetes. No wonder — it is the key to successful control of the disease. In fact, with more than half of the adult diabetics, diet can be the deciding factor in whether or not insulin or oral agents will be needed. Controlling excessive food intake lowers cholesterol and fat levels of the blood which may help prevent heart and vascular disease. For diabetics who need insulin, avoidance of overeating will prevent consistently elevated blood sugar levels which may cause lethargy, weakness, sleep disturbance, and several other more serious symptoms. In short, diet is crucial to proper diabetic control.

A common misconception is that diet implies either starvation or no variation whatsoever in foods eaten. I have seen diabetics so uninformed about the basics of diet and how it can be varied, and so concerned about keeping their blood sugars normal, that they rarely varied their diet. I knew one man, for instance, who ate the exact same breakfast, lunch, and dinner for over 30 years because he knew it kept his blood sugar in good control. Every day, he brought a banana, a thermos of milk, and a meatball sandwich with him on the road as he worked as a traveling salesman. He cooked the meatballs the night before to assure that he got the same amount of meat with the sandwich each day. Although he certainly did a good job controlling his blood sugar and was free of any major diabetic complications, I think he could have done just as well by spicing things up a bit

with a little variety! By knowing some basic nutritional information, food can be proportioned and varied so that ideal weight is
maintained, maximal strength is assured, blood sugar is controlled, and the taste buds are *satisfied!*

Knowing about food and diet is *not* restrictive. In fact, the
more you know about food, the *less* restrictive you have to be
with your daily schedule. By knowing the approximate caloric
intake of various foods, you will know how to adapt your nutritional needs to a schedule that suits you. You do not have to eat
supper at 5 PM or else . . . You can eat at 4 PM or 8 PM or any
other time as long as you know how to avoid hypoglycemia by
having an appropriate snack or making adjustments in insulin
dose. You can also decide which diet you prefer, be it vegetarian,
high-carbohydrate, or low-fat. When you dine at a restaurant,
you'll be able to choose from a menu with greater confidence.

What is the best way to learn about proper diet? One of the
worst ways is to use the so-called "free" diet. Too many people
interpret this diet as allowing one to eat *any* quantity of *any*
food that is available to munch on. With this misunderstanding,
caloric intake can range from 1200 to 4000, and the blood sugar
can range from 40 to 1000 mg%. The diabetics I have seen on
this diet simply don't do well. It is much safer to use the weighed
diet or the exchange diet, both of which will be discussed in this
section. By using either of these methods, you can get a good
idea of the approximate caloric intake of most foods. Food label-
ing has helped enormously in this regard and should be used as
an aid to diet planning. Once you know the approximate caloric
intake of the food you eat, you will be able to determine the
number of calories you need to get through the day and to keep
your weight ideal or get through a period of exercise. This
knowledge can help you avoid the unnecessary extremes in blood
sugar levels.

Before explaining in detail the exchange or weighed diet, it is
vital to know that every person is different metabolically, physically, and emotionally, and will thus need a different number of
calories per day than another person. It is educated guesswork
when a physician prescribes a certain number of calories for a
patient. Two thousand calories per day may prove to be too
much or too little for a particular person. In such a case, the

number of calories will have to be adjusted until the proper amount is determined. This proper amount will be known when the patient has achieved ideal weight and the blood sugar levels are controlled.

Understanding a diet depends on knowing some basic facts about nutrition. Let's review some useful information about food that can help you know whether you are getting the proper daily intake of vital nutrients. The following terms will be discussed:

1. gram
2. calorie
3. nutrient
4. Recommended Daily Allowance (RDA)
5. carbohydrates
6. proteins
7. fats
8. cholesterol
9. vitamins
10. fiber

1. Gram

A gram is a metric unit of weight. Approximately 30 grams equal one ounce.

2. Calorie

A calorie is a measurement of energy, scientifically defined as the amount of heat needed to raise one kilogram of water one degree Centigrade. Food contains calories in the form of carbohydrate, protein, fat, and alcohol. It has been determined that there are approximately 4 calories per gram of carbohydrate, 4 calories per gram of protein, 9 calories per gram of fat, and 7 calories per gram of alcohol. With this information and with the help of the federal program which has foods labeled according to their content of carbohydrate, protein, and fat, you should be able to calculate the number of calories in anything from a water bagel to a can of soup to a Pepperidge Farm cookie, and thus incorporate a wide variety of food into your daily diet.

3. Nutrient

A nutrient is a substance found in food that is essential for proper bodily function. Nutrients include carbohydrates, proteins, fats, water, minerals, and vitamins. An assortment of foods each day is essential for good nutrition.

4. Recommended Daily Allowance (RDA)

The U.S. Food and Nutrition Board has made recommendations based on studies of nutritional requirements of healthy men and women. From these studies, the Board has specified the necessary amounts of each nutrient for proper diet. It is important to remember that these recommendations are for healthy people. *Whether they are adequate for patients with poorly controlled diabetes is uncertain.*

5. Carbohydrates

Carbohydrates, often called the "fuel of life," are composed of three chemical elements: carbon, hydrogen, and oxygen. In an infinite number of combinations, these elements provide the major source of energy for most people of the world, particularly in Far Eastern countries where up to 80% of the diet is carbohydrate. Grown in fields and farm lands, carbohydrates are the least expensive energy source. They provide energy to all body cells, prevent the breakdown of body muscle and fat, and regulate water and mineral balance.

There are three classes of carbohydrates. The simplest form of carbohydrate is sugar. Sugars include table sugar, cane sugar, brown sugar, honey, raw or turbinado sugars. The sugars found in fruit (fructose) and milk (lactose) are also in this group.

The second group of carbohydrates is starch. Bread, cereal, pasta, tuber vegetables (such as potatoes, carrots, and turnips), and legumes (such as peas and beans) are all starches. During digestion, these starches are converted to sugar.

Cellulose is the third carbohydrate group. Cellulose includes stalks and leaves of vegetables, fruit skins, and seeds. As the most complex group of carbohydrates, cellulose cannot be digested in the human body, but it forms the necessary bulk for proper elimination.

6. Proteins

Proteins are nitrogen-containing compounds essential for life. They are made from simpler nitrogen-containing units called amino acids, of which there are 22 types. There are some amino acids that the human body must obtain from food because it cannot synthesize them. *Essential* amino acids are those that cannot be synthesized by the body.

All living cells contain protein. Protein is needed for growth, development, and tissue synthesis. It is interesting to note that insulin is a protein, as are other body hormones. The ability of the body to resist disease depends on "antibodies" which are also proteins.

The recommended daily allowance of protein is 56 grams for the average man and 46 for the average woman. The best source of protein is food of animal origin: milk, meat, poultry, and fish. All these sources provide the essential amino acids for human biological processes. For the vegetarian, legumes, grains, nuts, and vegetables should all be eaten daily to ensure adequate protein consumption.

7. Fats

Fats are a major energy source in food, containing 9 calories per gram, more than twice as many calories as carbohydrates or proteins. In America over 40% of the diet is comprised of fat.

Fat is necessary to help transport and absorb the fat-soluble vitamins A, D, E, and K. Fats are the principal storage form of calories and are very important in providing necessary energy during strenuous exercise.

Fats include *fatty acids, triglycerides, cholesterol,* and *lipoprotein.* Fatty acids are long carbon and hydrogen chains, called *hydrocarbons,* ending in a carbon, oxygen, and hydrogen unit called an *acid.* If all the carbons in the chain are filled with hydrogen, it is called a *saturated fat.* If hydrogen is missing from one of the carbons in the chain, it is called a *monounsaturated fat.* If hydrogen is missing from more than one carbon in the chain, it is called a *polyunsaturated fat.* Polyunsaturated fat lowers cholesterol levels, possibly by increasing fat excretion or decreasing synthesis. Fatty acids are the energy form used by the body when glucose is not available.

Triglycerides are combinations of a compound called *glycerol* with three fatty acids. Ninety percent of the body fat is contained in this form. When the blood level of triglycerides rises above 250 mg%, it is considered abnormally high, possibly a factor in heart disease.

8. Cholesterol

Cholesterol is a complex combination of fatty acids and a cyclic alcohol. It contributes to the formation of body hormones, vitamin D, and part of the bile. A high blood cholesterol level may be predisposing to heart disease. The level that is considered high and possibly dangerous is a major point of dispute among authorities. Certainly over 300 mg% is high, but I have seen some healthy 80-year-olds with these levels, so no definitive statement can be made about what levels are truly dangerous.

High density lipoprotein (HDL) is a complex fat and protein substance that has been the focus of much discussion in relation to cholesterol. Although HDL transports blood cholesterol throughout the body, it is thought to prevent cholesterol from lodging in the artery walls, thus preventing hardening of the arteries (arteriosclerosis). Exercise and a high fiber diet raise the HDL blood levels.

Low density lipoprotein (LDL) is also a fat and protein complex that transports cholesterol. However, whereas HDL may be very beneficial, LDL may, by an unknown mechanism, cause cholesterol to be released into arteries and therefore have more damaging effects, possibly accelerating arteriosclerosis.

9. Vitamins

Vitamins are a group of complicated substances found in small quantities in food which are *vital* to many bodily functions. At first, these substances were thought to be nitrogenous *(amines),* but since that time it has been learned that few vitamins are amines. The name "vitamin" still remains, however. Because the body cannot synthesize most vitamins, it must depend on dietary sources. There is a major controversy over the amount of vitamins needed for proper nutrition. Dr. Linus Pauling, the Nobel Prize-winning nuclear physicist, recommended high doses of vitamin C (over 2,000 mg/day!) for the prevention of the common cold. Most of the scientific community, however, does not believe this recommendation to be well-documented. It is generally believed that if there are adequate calories obtained using all the exchange lists, vitamin supplementation should not be needed. Below is a chart which lists the more common vitamins in terms of function, sources, and RDA.

	Function	Sources	RDA
Vitamin A	important for vision, skin integrity, and gland secretions; fights infection	green and yellow vegetables fruits	5,000 IU
Vitamin D	regulates absorption of calcium and phosphorus from the digestive tract; essential for bone development and preservation which will prevent fractures	fish milk	400 IU
Vitamin E	currently controversial; may protect red blood cells essential to cell respiration	vegetable oils margarine	15 IU
Vitamin K	necessary for blood clotting; may participate in energy transfer in tissues	fruits vegetables	not known
Vitamin C	necessary for supporting tissues and for healing wounds; important for many chemical reactions in cells, including the utilization of vitamins	fruits vegetables	45-70 mg
Thiamine (Vitamin B$_1$)	necessary for energy-generating activities, including proper use of oxygen, metabolism of glucose, and proper functioning of the central nervous system	bran wheat germ unmilled rice	1.2-2 mg

	Function	Sources	RDA
Riboflavin (Vitamin B$_2$)	constituent of body enzymes involved in metabolism of carbohydrate, protein, and fat	milk meat fish	1.2-2 mg
Niacin (Vitamin B$_3$)	constituent of body enzymes involved in metabolism of carbohydrate, protein, and fat	grains fish, meat peanuts wheat germ	18 mg
Pyridoxine (Vitamin B$_6$)	participates in enzyme systems; necessary for carbohydrate, protein, and fat metabolism	meat potatoes grains	1-2 mg
Vitamin B$_{12}$	necessary for proper function of all cells, metabolism of nerve cells, and utilization of fat, protein, and carbohydrate	animal protein, especially liver, muscle, meats, and dairy products	3-4 mg
Folic Acid	constituent of body enzymes needed for proper utilization of proteins and for formation of red blood cells and hemoglobin	leafy vegetables grains liver	400 mcg

10. Fiber

Over the past ten years, the importance of fiber in a well-balanced and nutritionally sound diet has come to the fore-ground. Fiber refers to the portion of vegetarian foods that cannot be digested by the stomach and intestines. It has been recommended that adults should get at least 25-40 grams of plant fiber per day. Whole grain products and certain vegetables (such as peas and beans) have a high content of plant fibers. Fruits are also a source of fiber, particularly fruits that are high in pectin (such as apples). Pectin has been shown to be helpful in lowering cholesterol levels. The benefits of fiber will be elucidated in the following discussion.

What is the Best Diet for the Diabetic?

When I developed diabetes in 1968, I was shocked by the amount of fat in the 2500 calorie ADA diet I was prescribed (which included eleven teaspoons of butter or the equivalent per day). It alarmed me because I knew that saturated fats and cholesterol are linked with cardiovascular disease, and that diabetics have a much higher incidence of high blood cholesterol, blood triglycerides, and associated vascular disease. In fact, it has been estimated that if it were not for deaths from heart attacks, non-insulin-dependent diabetics would live as long as nondiabetics.

Delving into this further, it became apparent to me why the diabetic diet was so traditionally high in fat. This dates back to the pre-insulin era when people with severe cases of diabetes could survive only on fat and possibly alcohol calories since carbohydrate calories tended to push the blood sugar level out of control. When insulin became available, carbohydrates were allowed in greater portions (although concentrated refined carbohydrates were still greatly restricted), but a large percent of the calories still came from fat. Only in the past few decades have we realized that the incidence of vascular disease is much higher with diabetics than with nondiabetics, possibly because of the traditional high-fat diet used by diabetics.

Furthermore, it has been discovered that there are other countries where not only is the incidence of diabetes lower, but the degree of vascular disease in the people who do have diabetes seems to be less severe when compared to the U.S. population. This is particularly true in Far Eastern and African countries where the diet tends to be high-fiber, high-carbohydrate, and low-fat.

Because of the traditionally high-fat diet and the high incidence of arteriosclerosis in American diabetics, several diabetic centers have experimented with a diet that is low in fat (less than 20% daily calories from fat), high in fiber (more than 40 grams daily), and high in carbohydrate (more than 60% daily calories from carbohydrate). Results were impressive, including improved blood sugar levels and lower cholesterol and triglyceride levels. Many patients were able to stop taking diabetes pills, and some patients could even discontinue their insulin injections.

Incidentally, the high-fiber content of the newer diets may have several other potential benefits for the diabetic. High-fiber diets have been helpful in treatment of colitis (spastic colon) and constipation. Colitis refers to the inflammation of the colon which may cause stomach or gas pains, and can be associated with bowel movement irregularity. Fiber apparently increases the bulk in the intestines and thereby keeps waste materials moving. Fiber in the diet is also believed to reduce incidence of colon cancer, perhaps indirectly by eliminating colitis.

Thus it would seem that the *best* diet for a diabetic may be a *high-fiber, high-carbohydrate,* and *low-fat* diet.

Meal Planning with Exchange Lists or with a Weighed Diet

In 1950 a committee of representatives from the American Diabetes Association, the American Dietetic Association, and the United States Public Health Service published a system of diet management. The proposed diet was based on a system of food groups or lists, called Exchange Lists.

An Exchange List consists of foods that have similar nutrient composition when used in a specified serving size. With exchanges, you can substitute one food for another within the same list. For example, 1/2 cup cooked string beans may be substituted for 1/2 cup carrots. However, a food in one exchange list should not be substituted for another; in other words, carrots should not be substituted for bacon.

When a diet is prescribed by a doctor, it is generally recommended that foods from each list be included so that all the necessary nutrients are consumed to provide energy and to regulate body functions. For example, if a diet consisted only of meat exchanges, the vitamin C and calcium content might be inadequate although the protein would be sufficient. Likewise, if only the bread and vegetable exchange lists were used, essential protein and vitamin B_{12} might be lacking.

I have modified the exchange list as proposed by the American Diabetes and Dietetic Associations by adding the gram weight for most of the foods presented. This approach gives even more exact information than the exchange list because it is more specific. For example, a "small" apple weighs approximately 80 grams.

Exchange Lists have been recently revised so that they now emphasize the use of foods containing lower levels of fat such as skim milk and lean meat. Certain vegetables are now included with the starches. The six Exchange Lists are as follows:

LIST ONE — Skim milk preferred. One exchange or 8 ounces contains 12 grams carbohydrate, 8 grams of protein, a trace of fat, and 80 calories. Whole milk, buttermilk, and other types of milk are also specified on the list.

LIST TWO — Vegetables. One exchange contains about 5 grams of carbohydrate, 2 grams of protein, 2 grams of fiber, and 25 calories. One exchange of a vegetable is 1/2 cup cooked or 120 grams. Some vegetables are more starchy and are included with the Bread Exchanges.

LIST THREE — Fruits. One exchange of fruit contains 10 grams of carbohydrate and 40 calories. Except for juices, fruits contain about 2 grams of fiber per exchange. Serving size depends on type of fructose (fruit sugar) which varies in different fruits.

LIST FOUR — Bread. This list includes bread, cereal, and *starchy* vegetables. One exchange contains 15 grams of carbohydrate, 2 grams of protein, and 70 calories. Several prepared foods fall into this category. Some bread exchanges are high in fiber.

LIST FIVE — Meat. One exchange of lean meat (1 ounce) contains 7 grams of protein, 3 grams of fat, and 55 calories. This list has been expanded, and choices can be made from meats and meat substitutes of various fat levels. Wise choices can reduce cholesterol intake.

LIST SIX — Fats. One exchange of fat contains 5 grams of fat and 45 calories. Here again, wise choices can be made to include polyunsaturated fats to help lower cholesterol levels.

An important thing to remember in diet planning is that your meal plan does not require many special foods or special food preparations. Foods used on the list are the same familiar foods purchased in your favorite supermarket. When you become familiar with the values that have been established for each food list and the type of food on each list, you will develop confidence in dealing with your diet. You will be able to dine at a new restaurant, the home of a friend, or even a fast food chain operation.

A federal program was initiated in 1973 which defined procedures to be used by food companies to specify the nutritive values of foods on product labels. With the expanded knowledge of your diet, you will be able to review new products and include them in your diet. The use of specially marked dietetic products is not always necessary nor recommended.

Remember, a diabetic diet is one you can live with. It can be reviewed, revised, or readjusted for special conditions such as pregnancy, hypertension, or high cholesterol levels. It can be adapted to a changed lifestyle or schedule. There are diet counselors available to help you when you need dietary advice. Use their services!

Good luck and good eating.

XIII
Food Exchange List
for Diabetics

Adapted from American Dietetic Association and
American Diabetes Association

1. MILK EXCHANGE

This list shows the kinds and amounts of milk or milk products to use for 1 Milk Exchange. The items in **boldface** are **nonfat**.

	Portion	Weight in Grams
Nonfat Fortified Milk:		
Skim or Nonfat Milk	1 cup	240
Powdered (nonfat dry, before adding liquid)	1/3 cup	25
Canned, Evaporated Skim Milk	1/2 cup	120
Buttermilk made from skim milk	1 cup	240
Yogurt made from skim milk (plain, unflavored)	1 cup	240
Lowfat Fortified Milk:		
1% Fat Fortified Milk (omit 1/2 Fat Exchange)	1 cup	240
2% Fat Fortified Milk (omit 1 Fat Exchange)	1 cup	240
Yogurt made from 2% fortified milk (plain, unflavored) (omit 1 Fat Exchange)	1 cup	240

1. MILK EXCHANGE (Continued)

	Portion	Weight in Grams
Whole Milk (omit 2 Fat Exchanges):		
Whole Milk	1 cup	240
Canned, Evaporated Whole Milk	1/2 cup	120
Buttermilk made from whole milk	1 cup	240
Yogurt made from whole milk (plain, unflavored)	1 cup	240

1 Milk Exchange equals 12 grams of carbohydrate, 8 grams of protein, a trace of fat, and 80 calories.

2. VEGETABLE EXCHANGE

Each 1/2 cup serving of the vegetables listed below counts as 1 Vegetable Exchange. Unless cooked with fat, all vegetables are **nonfat**. Asterisked vegetables are high in vitamin A.

Asparagus	Chilies
Bean Sprouts	Cucumbers
Beans, green or yellow	Eggplant
Beets	Mushrooms
Broccoli*	Okra
Brussels Sprouts	Onions
Cabbage	Peppers*
Carrots	Rhubarb
Cauliflower	Rutabaga
Celery	Sauerkraut

2. VEGETABLE EXCHANGE (Continued)

Spinach and Other Greens*   **Turnips***
Summer Squash   **Vegetable Juice Cocktail**
Tomatoes*   **Zucchini**
Tomato Juice

The following raw vegetables are all free exchanges and may be eaten in any amount:

> **Chicory*, Chinese Cabbage, Endive, Escarole, Lettuce, Parsley, Radishes, Watercress**

STARCHY VEGETABLES are found in the Bread Exchange List.

1 Vegetable Exchange equals 5 grams of carbohydrate, 2 grams of protein, 2 grams of fiber, and 25 calories.

3. FRUIT EXCHANGE

The amount of each fruit listed below (no sugar added) counts as 1 Fruit Exchange. Fruits are all **nonfat**. Asterisked fruits are high in vitamin C.

	Portion	Weight in Grams
Apple	1 small	80
Apple Juice or Cider	1/3 cup	100
Applesauce (unsweetened)	1/2 cup	120
Apricots (fresh)	2 medium	100
Apricots (dried)	4 halves	20
Banana	1/2 small	50
Berries		
Strawberries	3/4 cup	150
Other Berries	1/2 cup	120
Cherries	10 large	175
Dates	2	15
Figs (fresh or dried)	1	20
Grapefruit	1/2	125
Grapefruit Juice	1/2 cup	120
Grapes	12	75
Grape Juice	1/4 cup	60
Mango	1/2 small	70
Melon		
Cantaloupe*	1/4 small	200
Honeydew	1/8 medium	150
Watermelon	1 cup	175
Nectarine	1 small	100

3. FRUIT EXCHANGE (Continued)

	Portion	Weight in Grams
Orange*	1 small	100
Orange Juice*	1/2 cup	120
Papaya	3/4 cup	100
Peach	1 medium	100
Persimmon, native	1 medium	100
Pineapple	1/2 cup	80
Pineapple Juice	1/3 cup	80
Plums	2 medium	100
Prunes	2 medium	25
Prune Juice	1/4 cup	60
Raisins	2 tablespoons	15
Tangerine*	1 medium	100

Cranberries may be used as desired if no sugar is added.

1 Fruit Exchange equals 10 grams of carbohydrate, 2 grams of fiber (except for juices), and 40 calories.

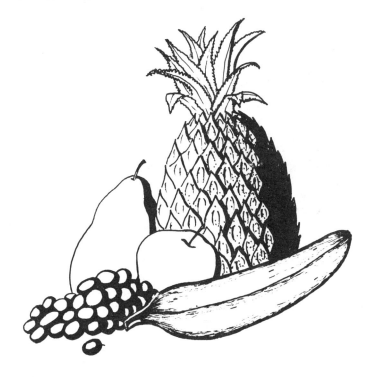

4. BREAD EXCHANGE

A serving of the following breads, cereals, starchy vegetables, and prepared foods counts as 1 Bread Exchange. The **boldfaced** items are **low-fat** Bread Exchanges. They have varying amounts of fiber.

	Portion	Weight in Grams
Bread:		
White, Whole Wheat,		
Rye, Pumpernickel,		
or Raisin	1 slice	25
Bagel, small	1/2	25
English Muffin, small	1/2	25
Plain Bread Roll	1	35
Frankfurter Roll	1/2	20
Hamburger Bun	1/2	20
Dried Bread Crumbs	3 tablespoons	20
Taco Shell	1	
Cereal:		
Bran Buds (high in fiber)	1/3 cup	20
Bran Flakes	1/2 cup	22
Other Ready-To-Eat		
Unsweetened Cereal	3/4 cup	25
Puffed Cereal		
(unfrosted)	1 cup	13
Cereal (cooked)	1/2 cup	100
Grits (cooked)	1/2 cup	100
Rice or Barley (cooked)	1/2 cup	75
Pasta (cooked)	1/2 cup	75
Popcorn (popped, no		
fat added)	3 cups	40
Cornmeal (dry)	2 tablespoons	
Flour	2½ tablespoons	
Wheat Germ	1/4 cup	28
Crackers:		
Arrowroot	3	20
Graham, 2½ inch	2	15
Matzo, 6 × 4 inch	1/2	20
Oyster	20	14
Pretzels, 3⅛ inch long,		
⅛ inch diameter	25	15
Rye Wafers, 3½ × 2 inch	3	15
Saltines	6	15
Soda, 2½ inch square	4	20

4. BREAD EXCHANGE (Continued)

	Portion	Weight in Grams
Dried Beans, Peas, and Lentils:		
Beans, Peas, Lentils (dried, cooked)	1/2 cup	100
Baked Beans, no pork (canned)	1/4 cup	50
Starchy Vegetables: (have 3-4 grams fiber per serving)		
Corn	1/3 cup	80
Corn on Cob	1 small	
Lima Beans	1/2 cup	90
Parsnips	2/3 cup	125
Peas, green (canned or frozen)	1/2 cup	90
Potato, white	1 small	100
Potato (mashed)	1/2 cup	100
Pumpkin	3/4 cup	
Winter Squash (cooked)	1/2 cup	100
Yam or Sweet Potato (cooked)	1/4 cup	50
Prepared Foods:		
Biscuit, 2-inch diameter (omit 1 Fat Exchange)	1	35
Corn Bread, 2 × 2 × 1 inch (omit 1 Fat Exchange)	1	35
Corn Muffin, 2-inch diameter (omit 1 Fat Exchange)	1	35
Crackers, round butter type (omit 1 Fat Exchange)	5	20
Muffin, plain small (omit 1 Fat Exchange)	1	40
Potatoes, French-fried (omit 1 Fat Exchange)	8	50
Potato or Corn Chips (omit 2 Fat Exchanges)	15	10

4. BREAD EXCHANGE (Continued)

	Portion	Weight in Grams
Pancake. 5 × 1/2-inch (omit 1 Fat Exchange)	1	45
Waffle, 5 × 1/2-inch (omit 1 Fat Exchange)	1	75

1 Bread Exchange equals 15 grams of carbohydrate, 2 grams of protein, 2 to 5 or more grams of fiber, and 70 calories.

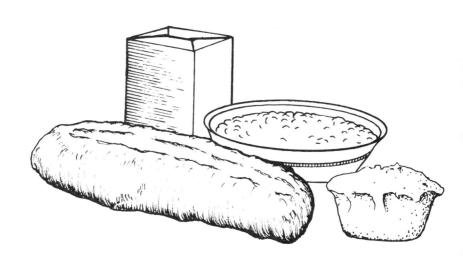

5. MEAT EXCHANGE

LEAN MEAT EXCHANGE

Each serving below is for cooked meat and counts as 1 Low-Fat Meat Exchange. All lean meats are **low in saturated fat and cholesterol**. These are preferable to other meat exchanges.

	Portion	Weight in Grams
Beef:		
Baby Beef (very lean), **Chipped Beef, Flank Steak, Tenderloin, Steaks (Sirloin and T-Bone,** trimmed), **Plate Ribs, Plate Skirt Steak** (round bottom, top), **All Cuts Rump, Tripe**	1 ounce	30
Lamb:		
Leg, Rib, Sirloin, Loin, Shank, Shoulder	1 ounce	30
Pork:		
Leg (whole rump, center shank), **Ham, Smoked** (center slices)	1 ounce	30
Veal:		
Leg, Loin, Rib, Shank, Shoulder, Cutlets	1 ounce	30
Poultry:		
Meat without skin of Chicken, Turkey, Cornish Hen, Guinea Hen, Pheasant	1 ounce	30
Fish:		
Any fresh or frozen	1 ounce	30
Canned Salmon, Tuna, Mackerel, Crab, Lobster	1/4 cup	
Clams, Oysters, Scallops, Shrimp	5 or 1 ounce	30
Sardines, drained	3	40

LEAN MEAT EXCHANGE (Continued)

	Portion	Weight in Grams
Cheeses, containing less than 5% butterfat	1 ounce	30
Cottage Cheese, dry and 2% butterfat	1/4 cup	60
Dried Beans and Peas (omit 1 Bread Exchange)	1/2 cup	100

1 Lean Meat Exchange equals 7 grams of protein, 3 grams of fat, and 55 calories.

MEDIUM-FAT MEAT EXCHANGE

Each serving listed below is for cooked meat and counts as 1 Medium-Fat Meat Exchange. Because of the additional fat in these items, charge yourself for both 1 Meat Exchange and 1/2 Fat Exchange for each Medium-Fat serving. The item listed in **boldface** is **low in saturated fat and cholesterol**.

	Portion	Weight in Grams
Beef: Ground (15% fat), Corned Beef (canned), Rib Eye, Round (ground, commercial)	1 ounce	30
Pork: Loin (all cuts Tenderloin), Shoulder Arm (picnic), Shoulder Blade, Boston Butt, Canadian Bacon, Boiled Ham	1 ounce	30
Variety Meat: Liver, Heart, Kidney, and Sweetbreads (high in cholesterol)	1 ounce	30
Cottage Cheese, creamed	1/4 cup	
Cheese: Mozzarella, Ricotta, Farmer's Cheese, Neufchatel	1 ounce	30
Parmesan	3 tablespoons	30
Egg (high in cholesterol)	1	30

MEDIUM-FAT MEAT EXCHANGE (Continued)

	Portion	Weight in Grams
Peanut Butter (omit 2 additional Fat Exchanges)	2 tablespoons	30

1 Medium-Fat Meat Exchange equals 7 grams of protein, 5.5 grams of fat, and 75 calories.

HIGH-FAT MEAT EXCHANGE

Each serving below is for cooked meat and counts as 1 High-Fat Meat Exchange. Because of the added fat content, charge yourself for both 1 Meat Exchange and 1 Fat Exchange for each High-Fat Meat Serving.

	Portion	Weight in Grams
Beef: Brisket, Corned Beef (Brisket), Ground Beef (more than 20% fat), Hamburger (commercial), Chuck (ground commercial), Roasts (Rib), Steaks (Club, Rib)	1 ounce	30
Lamb: Breast	1 ounce	30
Pork: Spareribs, Loin (Back Ribs), Pork (ground), Country-style Ham, Deviled Ham	1 ounce	30
Veal: Breast	1 ounce	30
Poultry: Capon, Duck (domestic), Goose	1 ounce	30
Cheddar Cheeses	1 ounce	30
Cold Cuts	4 ½ × ⅛-inch slice	30

HIGH-FAT MEAT EXCHANGE (Continued)

	Portion	Weight in Grams
Frankfurter	1 small	30

1 High-Fat Meat Exchange equals 7 grams of protein, 8 grams of fat, and 100 calories.

6. FAT EXCHANGE

Foods that appear in **boldface** are **polyunsaturated**.

	Portion	Weight in Grams
Margarine, soft, tub or stick*	1 teaspoon	5
Margarine, regular stick	1 teaspoon	5
Avocado, 4-inch diameter**	1/8	25
Butter	1 teaspoon	5
Bacon Fat	1 teaspoon	5
Bacon (crisp-cooked)	1 strip	10
Cream (light or sour)	2 tablespoons	30
Cream (heavy)	1 tablespoon	15
Cream Cheese	1 tablespoon	15
French or Italian Dressing***	1 tablespoon	15
Lard	1 teaspoon	5
Mayonnaise***	1 teaspoon	5
Nuts:		
Almonds*	10 whole	10
Pecans*	2 large whole	10
Peanuts*		
Spanish	20 whole	15
Virginia	10 whole	15
Walnuts	6 small	8
Other*	6 small	10

*Made with corn, cottonseed, safflower, soy, or sunflower oil only.

**Fat content is primarily monounsaturated.

***If made with corn, cottonseed, safflower, soy, or sunflower oil, can be used on fat-modified diet.

6. FAT EXCHANGE (Continued)

	Portion	Weight in Grams
Oil:		
Corn, Cottonseed, Safflower, Soy, Sunflower, Olive**, Peanut**	1 teaspoon	5
Olives**	5 small	
Salad Dressing, mayonnaise type***	2 teaspoons	10
Salt Pork	3/4-inch cube	

**Fat content is primarily monounsaturated.

***If made with corn, cottonseed, safflower, soy, or sunflower oil, can be used on fat-modified diet.

1 Fat Exchange equals 5 grams of fat and 45 calories.

There are some foods that you won't find on the exchange lists. Salt, pepper, herbs, spices, parsley, lemon, horseradish, vinegar, mustard, celery salt, onion salt or powder, garlic, and bottled hot pepper sauce are all flavor bonuses with a "free" exchange rating. Diet calorie-free beverages, tea, coffee, nonfat bouillon, unsweetened gelatin, and unsweetened pickles are free, too.

Also, there are *quick energy foods* containing sugar that may be needed from time to time to treat low sugar reactions or prevent them. A list of these foods with the approximate amount of sugar in each is listed on the following page.

QUICK ENERGY FOOD LIST

Food	Portion	Bread Exchange	Fat Exchange	Fruit Exchange
Date Bar	1 (2 × 1-inch)	1/2	1	
Animal Crackers	8	1		
Bisco Sugar Wafers	6	1	1	
Chocolate Covered Grahams	2	1	1	
Chocolate Fudge Cookie Break Creme Sandwich	2	1	1	
Creme Wafer Sticks	3	1	1	
Fig Newton Cakes	2	1		
Oatmeal Cookies	1½	1		
Old Fashioned Ginger Snaps	3	1		
Oreo Creme Sandwich	2	1	1	
Vanilla Wafers	5	1		
Apple Danish Coffee Cake 14 oz.	1/8	1/2	2	1

The following chart is a guide showing the approximate number of each of the various exchanges that should be included in the daily diet. Note that the number of exchanges varies according to the daily caloric intake that is allowed. The figures have been rounded to the nearest whole number. Other arrangements are possible and plans may be modified to suit individual preferences or needs. In general, the exchanges should be spread out in three to six meals. Three is better for the non-insulin-dependent diabetic and six is better for the insulin-dependent diabetic.

Calories	Carbo-hydrates	Protein	Fat	Milk	Vege-tables	Fruit	Bread	Meat	Fat
	Grams			Exchanges					
800	85	55	27	1	3	3	2	5	2
1000	100	70	38	1	3	3	3	7	3
1200	125	85	41	2	3	3	3	7	3
1400	145	90	51	2	3	3	6	7	5
1500	160	95	54	2	3	3	6	9	5
1800	215	105	59	3	3	6	7	9	6
2000	245	110	64	3	3	6	9	9	7
2400	260	150	86	3	3	6	10	14	9

XIV
How to Use the Exchange Diet System

For Diabetics Not on Insulin

S UPPOSE you have a weight problem along with your diabetes, and your doctor prescribes a diet of approximately
1200 calories. Because this particular doctor is hard-pressed for
time, he simply gives you a diet list, wishes you luck, directs you
to the exit door, and expects you to know what to do from there.
This lack of explanation may mean the end of the diet (and
understandably so!) before it ever begins.

However, now that you understand more about nutrition and
food exchanges, you can take the bull by the horns, gather relevant information, and create your own meal plan within the lim-
its the doctor has outlined for you. Using the exchange chart,
you find that for a 1200-calorie diet you are allowed the following
exchanges: 2 milk, 3 vegetable, 3 fruit, 3 bread, 7 meat, and 3 fat.
By checking your cupboards, refrigerator, and wallet, and by
knowing what foods are most appealing to you, you can satisfy
your hunger and your creative impulses by designing a meal
plan that suits you and incorporates the exchanges you are
allowed. Your plan might look something like the table on the
following page.

You will notice that this sample meal plan provides no
between-meal snacks. Theoretically, it may be better to eat nutritional snacks between meals and eat less food for breakfast,
lunch, and dinner so that less insulin from the pancreas is

required at any given time to assimilate the food. However, by eating between the three traditional daily meals, there is further titillation of the taste buds, and there is a greater chance of succumbing to the deadly sin of gluttony. Therefore, if you have a difficult time controlling your appetite, three meals per day may be preferable.

	Milk	Vegetable	Fruit	Bread	Meat	Fat
Breakfast	1/2 cup skim milk; 1/2 cup with cereal		3/4 cup straw-berries	20 grams or 2/3 ounce Bran Buds	1/2 cup cottage cheese	
Lunch	iced tea	lettuce	1 medium peach (100 grams)	1 slice rye bread	3 ounces or 90 grams ham	1 tsp mayon-naise
Dinner	8 ounces skim milk	salad and 1/2 cup beets	1/4 canta-loupe (200 grams)	1/3 cup corn (80 grams)	3 ounces hamburger	1 tsp salad dressing

Once you are on your diet for a given length of time (perhaps four to six weeks), you will know if you are succeeding by checking your weight and blood sugar. Depending on how well you are faring, you can add or subtract 100 to 300 calories from your daily intake for another four- to six-week period. REMEMBER: Patience and stick-to-it-iveness provide a winning strategy. Quick-loss fad diets have had little lasting success. Weight loss takes time since it took time for your unwanted pounds to accumulate. Stick to it and don't become frustrated!

This brings me to one final point. What happens if you *do* succumb and eat some tempting delicacy or, as my patients say, "cheat?" When this happens, I implore you not to give up, for you are not alone. In fact, you are probably in the majority. In my extensive practice with diabetics, I know very few people who do not slip off their diet from time to time. The major point is to be as conscientious as you can without giving up if your will power takes a temporary nose dive. One splurge in and of itself will not smash your progress and goals.

I know one person who actually sets aside a certain time during the week to snack on a particular goodie. By this *controlled* indulgence (the words are not necessarily mutually exclusive!) you may be more likely to stick to your diet during the rest of the week. Dieting is *not* a punishment! Instead, it is self-awareness and modification of habits for a healthier you.

For Insulin-Dependent Diabetics

If you require insulin injections for diabetic control, you can use diet guidelines similar to those described for the non-insulin-dependent diabetic. There are a few distinctions, however. While the non-insulin-dependent diabetic can usually choose between three moderate or six light meals per day, it is better for you to eat the six smaller meals per day so that there is not such a time lapse between meals, especially when you are active. A non-insulin-dependent diabetic can often skip meals without seriously risking hypoglycemia, but if you as an insulin-dependent diabetic skip meals, the risk of hypoglycemia is much greater. If you do find that you can skip a meal without developing hypoglycemia, it may be because your blood glucose is very high at the time so that it takes several hours to reduce it to normal levels. Although skipping a meal may help normalize blood levels, it is *much* better not to have elevated blood sugar in the first place!

Another major problem you may experience is how to reduce caloric intake when you are taking so much insulin. I have often seen insulin-dependent diabetics consume way too many calories and then take a large dose of insulin to keep the blood glucose from getting exceedingly high. Then, when the doctor says to cut back on the calories, the diabetic will complain that when he does so, he feels weak and uncomfortable. The explanation is that the pateint is suffering from hypoglycemia due to the calorie cutback while he is still taking a relatively large amount of insulin.

If you have been in a similar predicament, the best thing to do is to cut back on calories *gradually* (perhaps by 100 calories or so every 2 to 3 days) while at the same time gradually reducing your insulin dose (maybe by 2 to 4 units). This is another situation where home blood sugar monitoring is a useful guide in determining how much to decrease the calories and insulin dose without developing hypoglycemia. Your doctor should be able to answer any questions you may have about modification of calorie intake or insulin dose.

XV
Weight Loss

Eat little and avoid sweets.
— *Leo Tolstoy in his Ten Rules of Life*

No one ever regrets having eaten too little.
— *Thomas Jefferson*

How to get thin — do not eat bread, cake, potatoes, rice, cream, butter, milk, pastries, sweets, fats, minces, puddings, stews, saltmeats, fish, or anything containing starch or *sugar!*
— *General George Patton*

IN 50% of the cases of overweight diabetics, weight loss is critical in controlling diabetes. In these cases, shedding excess pounds will help lower blood sugars to normal levels or at least improve them enough so that insulin or oral agents may not be necessary. Yet many patients faced with a weight problem say despondently, "All I have to do is *look* at food and I gain weight." Many of these patients will go to their doctors with their weight problems and will be accused of not following their diet correctly, with the implication that they are lying if they say they do. As a result, they become further depressed with their lack of results (as well as with their looks) and give up completely.

The reasons why some patients have so much difficulty losing weight are complex. It is probably true that some people can eat more than others and not have a weight problem. For instance, women patients sometimes say, "My husband eats twice as much as I do and he is as skinny as a rail." The explanation for this probably lies in the difference in body chemistry and hormones, but medical research still has no definitive explanation.

Be this as it may, how do patients lose weight? Many books have been written which advocate the low-carbohydrate diet. True, many patients lose weight on this diet, but it is frequently "water weight" and as soon as they begin eating many starches again, which they inevitably do, they rapidly gain back much of the weight they had lost.

Furthermore, a low-carbohydrate diet may be quite dangerous. Frequently, people who indulge in a heavy amount of physical exercise will feel weak, tired, or sick while on these diets. More seriously, they may be susceptible to acidosis, especially if they include alcohol in their diet. A low-carbohydrate diet may also make people more prone to low blood pressure and mineral deficiencies, especially low potassium. Death itself has been attributed to low-carbohydrate diets. For these reasons, diabetics should not follow these diets unless they are under the close supervision of a physician.

The only way for patients to lose weight is to consume fewer calories than their bodies burn. They must determine the optimum number of calories per day that will cause a weight loss. They must then adhere as closely as possible to that figure.

The realization that obesity is not just a cosmetic problem, but a health problem as well, is the first step toward a successful weight loss program. Weight Watchers and Overeaters Anonymous are two organizations that have been very successful in overcoming the psychological barriers of losing weight. Psychoanalysis, psychotherapy, and hypnosis are expensive alternatives that may also be helpful. Behavior modification has also become popular for many patients with weight problems. This program identifies several situations and moods for which the response of overeating has become almost automatic. Watching television, working in the kitchen, attending social events, and being bored or depressed after a long day are factors which frequently cause overeating. By keeping a diary of daily events and connecting these events to food eaten, patients may learn what prompts them to overeat, and they may learn to avoid the circumstances that trigger the overeating.

Knowledge of caloric and nutrient value of foods is also a great aid in weight control. Many patients are unaware of the number of calories contained in the foods they eat. Sweets are frequently higher in fat calories than in sugar calories. Nuts, seeds, and fried foods are especially high in calories because of their fat content. It is important, then, to limit the intake of these high-fat foods as well as those containing sugar calories.

As will be discussed in the next chapter, another strategy to help shed those extra pounds is to make the body burn more calories; in other words, exercise more. If the body burns an extra 500 calories per day, half a pound or more per week will be lost.

Marathoners exemplify the art of weight control. Besides exercising regularly, they tend to follow more nutritious diets, eliminating "junk" food and desserts. This high-exercise, low-junk-food regimen certainly seems to pay off, for it is very rare to see an overweight marathoner.

XVI

The Glycemic Index and the Sweet Tooth

IN the summer of 1983, an article in one of the most prestigious medical journals, *The New England Journal of Medicine,* indicated that plain sugar caused no more a rise in blood sugar — in nondiabetics and diabetics alike — than did an equal caloric equivalent of potato or wheat starch. The daily newspapers interpreted this to mean that some diabetics can eat sugar. This was very welcome news indeed for those diabetics who have the same weakness as nondiabetics for foods that have been made especially enticing by the addition of various sugars or sweeteners.

The medical community, however, was stunned, having long believed in the value of distinguishing between simple and complex carbohydrates. The simple ones were the sugars like sucrose, glucose, and fructose which caused immediate rise in blood sugar, while the complex ones, such as potatoes and whole grain bread, caused much less blood sugar rise. Well, *The New England Journal of Medicine* article was not the only one to bring this dogma into doubt. Other recent studies have reached similar conclusions, indicating that foods of equal caloric value may have differing tendencies to raise blood sugar and that the determining factor was *not* whether the foods were made of simple or complex carbohydrates. This tendency of foods to raise blood sugar is measured by a system now referred to as the "glycemic index," which uses glucose as the food against which all others are measured since glucose has the greatest tendency to raise blood sugar.

Some of the responses of blood sugar to various foods were printed in *American Health,* January/February 1984, and are shown below. As you can see from this chart, fructose, the simple sugar found in many fruits and vegetables, has a relatively low glycemic index, causing much less of a rise in blood sugar than equivalent calories in potato or cereal. Peanuts also produce a very low blood sugar response, although their large fat content makes them a snack to be wary of, especially if body weight and blood cholesterol are problems.

WHICH FOODS BOOST INSULIN? This list shows how quickly different foods boost blood sugar and raise your insulin. Foods with a high number act the most like glucose, leading to an insulin jump. Foods with a low index give a slow rise in blood sugar — fructose, fruits, complex carbohydrates.

Honey and Sugars

Fructose	20	Honey	87
Sucrose	59	Glucose	100

Bread, Pasta, Corn and Rice

Whole-wheat spaghetti	42	Brown rice	66
		White bread	69
White spaghetti	50	Wheat bread	72
		White rice	72
Sweet corn	59		

Breakfast Cereals

Oatmeal	49	Shredded Wheat	67
All-bran	51	Cornflakes	80

Fruits

Apples	39	Bananas	62
Oranges	40	Raisins	64
Orange juice	46		

Root Vegetables

Sweet potatoes	48	White potatoes	70
Yams	51	Carrots	92
Beets	64	Parsnips	97

Dairy Products

Skim milk	32	Ice cream	36
Whole milk	34	Yogurt	36

Peas and Beans

Soybeans	15	Chickpeas	36
Lentils	29	Lima beans	36
Kidney beans	29	Baked beans	40
Black-eyed peas	33	Frozen peas	51

Odds and Ends

Peanuts	13	Sponge cake	46
Sausages	28	Potato chips	51
Fish sticks	38	Pastry	59
Tomato soup	38	Mars bar	68

This brings up some crucial points, for these studies knock at the very foundation of the ADA Exchange System that has been recommended for years. They may, however, help to explain why some diabetics have found their blood sugar 120 mg% on one day and 240 mg% the next, frustrated by the fact that they had not "cheated" on their exchange diets; the answer may lie in their having eaten foods of the same caloric value but differing glycemic index value, e.g., an apple versus a banana, orange juice versus an orange.

These studies also seem to be somewhat conflicting with the high-fiber, low-fat diets of Nathan Pritikin and James Anderson, M.D., as some studies have shown that whole wheat bread tends to cause more of a rise in blood sugar than does ice cream. Pritikin and Anderson have done tremendous work with their diet and exercise programs helping many people with diabetes and vascular disorders. However, their diets curtail a great deal of fat, and while it may be that the fat and caloric intake of the average American is more detrimental than the sugar intake, it is also very possible that diabetics do not have to be quite as restrictive of the simple carbohydrates as Pritikin and Anderson recommend. If this turns out to be true, the Exchange System will have to be revamped to incorporate the newer information on the glycemic index. More studies are required to examine this concept more fully.

Finally, this brings up a key question that is constantly being bandied about among people in the health fields: Should diabetics eat sweets? There are some foods with sweeteners that have no calories in them, such as cyclamate, saccharin, and the newer one, aspartame, which is derived from protein. These should have little effect on blood sugar and therefore can be consumed without fear. Reasons not to consume them might be the taste, especially bitter in saccharin, and the cost. (Aspartame sweeteners tend to be higher in cost.) There is some concern that cyclamate and saccharin may cause cancer, but studies that have been done over the past ten years have *not* shown an increased incidence of cancer in saccharin users. Average consumption of such sweeteners is probably quite safe.

As for the caloric sweeteners, there are several on the market. They may contain table sugar (sucrose), glucose (dextrose), fructose (fruit sugar), or sorbitol. Sorbitol is closely related in composition to glucose and fructose. The amount of sorbitol a person can eat is probably somewhat limited because an excessive amount causes a disturbing bout of diarrhea. Regardless, care should be taken not to overdo any of these sweets.

While it is probably quite true that cake or candy will not cause more of a rise in blood sugar than an equal number of calories from white potato or bread, it is also true that especially rich cake, such as Chocolate Mousse de Quoi, frequently has extra calories from butter, fat, or protein, so that the intake has to be a very small quantity in order to avoid going overboard. There are not many mortals who can limit themselves to such a miniscule portion of such an enticing sweet. The temptation to overindulge is simply too great, even for well-disciplined diabetics, and especially if they are placing too much confidence in the new glycemic index theory. Many diabetics who must watch their caloric intake to keep their weight, as well as blood sugar, down might also be tempted to sacrifice nutritious foods just to have that high-calorie piece of cake. By eating sweets from table sugar, more insulin is needed to keep the blood sugar normal, and insulin per se may further provoke the appetite and then more overeating, thus setting up a vicious cycle. If, despite all good intentions, they are still inclined to incorporate a small amount of sweets in their diet, it is imperative to test their blood sugars to see the response. They may especially want to try some confections that are made with fructose to prove for themselves what many of the studies alluded to above seem to have shown (i.e., that fructose has a low glycemic index).

Overweight Type II diabetics who suffer from high blood insulin levels should be particularly interested in how the body responds to various types of sugars. As reported by Dr. Judith Rodin, professor of psychology at Yale, in the January/February 1984 issue of *American Health,* fructose may not stimulate the appetite as much as glucose. In her study, she found that when volunteers were given a drink with 192 calories from fructose in it, they subsequently ate much less compared to volunteers who were given a 192-calorie glucose drink. She believes this is because fructose causes much less triggering of blood insulin and consequently less triggering of the appetite.

Conclusion and Recommendation

Recent work has surprised many by showing that foods of the same caloric value provoke dissimilar rises in blood sugar, due to differing "glycemic indices." Ice cream, for example, may cause less of a rise in blood sugar than whole wheat bread. Despite these recent findings, I would be cautious about indulging in sweets for the above-explained reasons, and I would definitely continue to rely on blood sugar testing, keeping in mind that the ideal goal is to keep the blood sugar as close to the 60-120 mg% range as possible.

XVII
The Power of Exercise

Socrates: And is not bodily habit spoiled by rest
and idleness, but preserved for a long
time by motion and exercise?
— *Plato*, Theaetetus

THE value of exercise in medicine has been debated over the years. Controversy still reigns over whether exercise really does help prevent heart attacks, hypertension, and strokes. Diabetes has not been free of this controversy. In fact, for many years, exercise for the diabetic was considered by many physicians to be strictly *verboten*. Children with diabetes were considered sickly and were pampered and isolated from their sports-minded friends. The psychological consequences of this attitude included depression and rebellion. Fortunately, there has been a shift in attitude during recent years, and the value of exercise for the diabetic has been more fully recognized.

We owe thanks to people like Bill Talbert, the outstanding U.S. champion tennis professional, who has been taking insulin since shortly after its discovery in the 1920s. The hockey player Bobby Clark developed diabetes at age 14 and went on to score over 1000 points in the National Hockey League. He was voted Most Valuable Player several times. Other diabetic sports stars include Jackie Robinson, Catfish Hunter, and Ron Santo. At last, we know that exercise need not be eliminated or curtailed from a diabetic's lifestyle. Diabetics can be highly capable of strenuous exercise and outstanding sports achievements. This is

no more evident than in the stellar performance of Pete Powers
(now a physician) who has had diabetes since age 14 and has
run a marathon in a speedy 2 hours and 42 minutes!

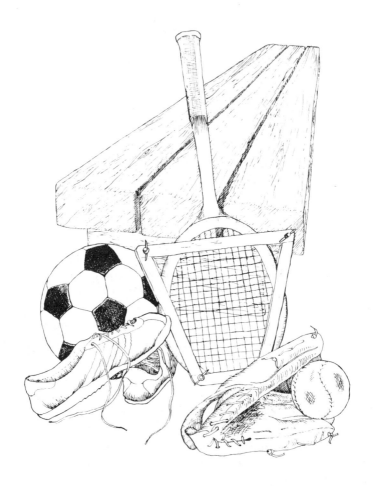

Nowhere in medicine is the effect of exercise as profound as
it is in diabetes. Particularly in insulin-dependent diabetics,
exercise can have a dramatic effect in lowering blood sugar levels if the diabetes is well controlled. In children diabetics' camps,
where exercise is emphasized heavily, the average insulin dose
of the campers can often be halved with no change in diet.

Although the effect of exercise may differ somewhat between the insulin-dependent and non-insulin-dependent diabetic, exercise usually allows a diabetic to eat more while maintaining normal blood sugar levels.

Exercise for the Insulin-Dependent Diabetic

To understand the effect of exercise, it is important to remember that diabetics have a disturbed insulin mechanism which must be compensated for in order to benefit from exercise without developing hypoglycemia. This is especially true for the insulin-dependent diabetic whose pancreas secretes little or no insulin.

In the nondiabetic, the blood insulin level drops with exercise, thereby allowing blood sugar levels to remain within the normal range. In the insulin-dependent diabetic, the blood insulin level depends on the amount and type of insulin injected and the rate with which it is absorbed. In addition, the absorption rate of insulin may depend on the type of exercise and the site of injection, i.e., whether the site is arm, stomach, or leg. When the diabetic is at rest, insulin is absorbed more quickly in the arm than in the leg. However, when the legs are used in exercise, insulin is absorbed more quickly, and if insulin is injected there, it may have a more drastic effect on the blood sugar level and an insulin reaction could occur.

Besides the more rapid absorption of insulin from the injection site, the fact that exercise increases the effect of insulin also has to be considered in order to prevent blood sugar levels that are too high or too low. There are variable factors that only the diabetic can estimate, such as how rigorous the exercise, how tough the opponent, and duration of the exercise.

Depending on all of the factors mentioned above, blood insulin levels can fluctuate, causing the blood sugar level to drop too low, stay within normal range, or go higher as in the case of many poorly controlled diabetics. For the sports-minded diabetic, especially the competitive one, the level of blood sugar can be a critical factor in performance. Most diabetic athletes seem to agree that high blood sugar levels result in less than optimum performance and that low blood sugar levels may result in poor performance as well as embarrassment, such as confusion on the basketball court resulting in points for the opposition.

From this discussion it becomes apparent that in order to control diabetes while exercising, an appropriate change in insulin or extra food may be needed. To help determine the necessary adjustments, a sensitive urine test method (such as *Tes-Tape*) or home blood sugar tests (such as *Chemstrip bG*) may be helpful. If it is determined that the blood sugar level is low or normal, extra food before and/or during a period of extended or rigorous exercise is probably wise. The type of food depends on the kind of exercise and when it is performed. For instance, a boxer might consume a form of concentrated sugar such as one or two packs of Lifesavers since he does not want a full stomach, but a marathon runner may consume sugar, liquids, or possibly both before and during exercise. In addition, most diabetic athletes prefer to reduce the amount of insulin taken before a period of extended exercise to reduce the risk of an insulin reaction. For brief periods of exercise, such as sprints or light tennis doubles, no alteration in insulin or food is usually necessary.

It is impossible for the diabetic's doctor to know exactly how to adjust the insulin dose or food intake to compensate for a period of exercise. Here again, as emphasized throughout this book, the patient must often be his own doctor, estimating how much exercise he has done, the calories burned, and whether the insulin injection site is a factor in the rate of insulin absorption. Then, with the help of a sensitive urine test or a self blood sugar test, an appropriate adjustment in insulin or diet can be made if necessary.

The following table indicates the *approximate* number of calories expended per hour for various activities. The calories will vary according to body weight, air temperature, and the vigor with which the individual exercises. This table should prove helpful to both the insulin-dependent and non-insulin-dependent diabetic in determining how to make necessary adjustments for exercise.

Exercise for the Non-Insulin-Dependent Diabetic

For the non-insulin-dependent diabetic, exercise is also helpful in lowering both the blood sugar levels and the resistance to insulin that many non-insulin-dependent diabetics experience. As discussed earlier, non-insulin-dependent diabetics have fewer

Activity	Calories Burned Per Hour
Sleeping	40–80
Eating	50–90
Dishwashing	70–150
Walking	100–200
Housecleaning	120–300 or more
Dancing	150–300
Bicycling	150–300 or more
Golf (cart vs walking)	150–300 or more
Tennis (singles vs doubles)	200–600 or more
Horseback Riding	250–400
Ice Skating	250–400
Racquetball	300–600
Swimming	300–600
Skiing	400–800
Jogging:	
4 mph	360–420
5 mph	480–600
6 mph	600–750
over 6 mph	600–1000 or more

insulin receptors on the body cells, which is why there seems to be a resistance to insulin. It has been shown that regular and rigorous exercise can markedly increase the number of functioning receptors, and less insulin is therefore needed. This can be true even if the diabetic does not lose weight. (Weight loss is another factor that lowers the resistance to the effect of insulin.) Since exercise accelerates weight loss as well, the improvement in diabetes is that much more magnified. Thus, not as much insulin is needed by the pancreas. Non-insulin-dependent diabetics should heed the advice of the long distance runner who, when asked why he ran 1000 miles per year, said, "I am preserving my pancreas."

Other Effects of Exercise

Besides lowering blood sugar levels, exercise may aid weight reduction by burning more calories and lowering the blood levels of cholesterol and triglycerides. Exercise may also raise levels of HDL (the substance found in the blood which may prevent heart disease), increase longevity by preventing or reducing the severity of heart attacks, and improve hypertension. In addition, exercise for 30 minutes or more, several times per week, will make diabetics and nondiabetics alike feel better both physically and mentally. Although fatigued and depressed prior to exercise, many experience increased strength and heightened spirits during and after exercise. For all of these reasons, "EXERCISE IS POWER." If possible, it should be tried.

Caution

Despite the many excellent reasons to exercise, some diabetics should be cautious and should probably obtain their physician's advice before beginning an exercise program. This is especially true of adult-onset diabetics who have heart disease but may not be aware of it. For some reason, these diabetics may not experience typical heart symptoms which would alert them that heart disease is present. For these patients and for those who know they have heart disease, a good physical examination and a stress electrocardiogram (an exercise heart test) is recommended before beginning an exercise program.

For patients with eye disease, especially proliferative retinopathy, exercise may aggravate their condition. Exercise increases blood pressure during the exercise period and may cause eye bleeding in patients with proliferative retinopathy. (See the discussion of retinopathy in the chapter entitled "Complications.") A diabetic, even if he has no vision problem, should have an eye check at least once a year to make sure retinopathy is not present.

Other diabetics who should exercise with caution are those with decreased blood flow to their legs and those with neuropathy. These diabetics should be extremely careful not to get blisters which could become infected. If they have impaired circulation, they may not be able to get enough blood to the exercising muscle.

The Doctor at Sport

As you read this section on exercise, you may wonder how this wise doctor/author handles himself when *he* is exercising. Does he ever get into trouble? As a matter of fact, I *did* get into trouble very recently. I was initially displaying outstanding athletic skill by building up a 6-0, 3-0 tennis lead against one of my arch rivals. Suddenly, I was overcome by weakness, my legs began to wobble, my tennis strokes fell short, my concentration plummeted, and the score quickly took a turn for the worse to 3-4.

Fortunately, my wife was nearby and watching the sudden change of events. Hinting that my sugar must be low, she offered me a Coke. Thank heaven! Voraciously, I gulped it down. The sugar quickly seeped into my bloodstream and energized me. My tennis opponent, who was temporarily beaming with the thought of a likely comeback, again became despondent as my serves smashed in, my speed returned, my volleys were crisp and accurate, and my concentration was keen. The game was over for my flabbergasted opponent and I need not tell you the score.

Although this story may exaggerate my tennis ability, it does illustrate the point that it is very difficult to know exactly what your blood sugar is in the throes of exercise. The intensity and duration of the exercise can make all the difference in the world, possibly causing radical shifts in sugar levels. For this reason, quick energy foods should be within easy reach to treat hypoglycemia, should it occur. Don't be embarrassed to carry a carbohydrate with you or to make sure it can be easily obtained. Someone should know you are a diabetic, be it your opponent, partner, teammate, or spectator, so that he or she can remind you to take sugar in case the mental concentration of competitive sport makes it slip your mind. Advise your sport colleagues on the use of glucagon as discussed in the chapter on hypoglycemic reactions.

Exercise is not an insulin substitute for the insulin-dependent diabetic, but it does make diabetes easier to control. And since less insulin is needed, the cost of insulin treatment is less. Although there have been no well-documented studies to prove it, I firmly believe that diabetics who exercise fare much better physically and emotionally than those who don't. As a diabetic who jogs regularly over 650 miles per year and who plays competitive tennis, I am convinced that exercise is critical in achieving good diabetic control.

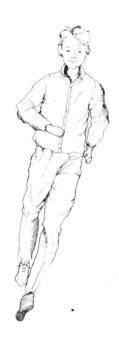

XVIII

Diabetes and the Woman: Pregnancy and the Menses

Pregnancy

A MONG physicians, there is almost universal agreement that the closer to normal that blood sugars are maintained during pregnancy, the better the outcome. Even for the nondiabetic mother, pregnancy is not easy due to discomfort, weight gain, and a tendency towards problems such as varicose veins and bladder infection. But for the woman with diabetes, pregnancy also means paying very strict attention to diet and insulin intake (if insulin is needed) and, in some cases, sharply limiting her activities.

Thanks to present-day medical management, the chances of a successful pregnancy in the diabetic woman now closely parallel those of the nondiabetic woman. Twenty years ago, however, this was not the case. Babies of diabetic women were then faced with a high risk of mortality. The improvement that has occurred over the past few decades has resulted from improved diabetic control and better methods of determining when delivery should occur.

Pregnancy causes dramatic bodily changes in a woman. One effect of pregnancy is a marked change in a woman's hormonal output, usually after the third month, after which sugar is not utilized as efficiently. Another effect is that the placenta produces hormones that block the effect of insulin. These hormonal changes sometimes trigger the development of diabetes in a previously nondiabetic woman. This condition is called *pregnancy diabetes*. For some women the diabetes will disappear once pregnancy is over, but for others the diabetes may be permanent.

For the woman who is diabetic prior to pregnancy, the changes associated with pregnancy lead to increased difficulty in controlling the diabetes. In the early stage of pregnancy, "morning sickness" may occur, possibly associated with decreased food intake. At the same time, the uterus and developing baby may be using more calories! As a result, it is possible that the diabetic woman may need less insulin during the first two to three months of pregnancy. It is very important to monitor both the caloric and insulin intake during this period to avoid the risk of insulin reactions.

As pregnancy continues, hormones are produced which block the effect of insulin and create a tendency towards high blood sugar. As a result, it is common to need more than twice as much insulin later in pregnancy in order to get blood sugar in the near-normal range and to *keep* it there. High blood sugar strains the fetal pancreas and may produce high blood insulin levels in the fetus. These factors may result in "big babies" or create respiratory problems and other complications in the newborn, including hypoglycemia.

It is clear that maintaining normal blood sugars is the way to ensure the best possible outcome of the pregnancy. How is this accomplished? By controlling blood sugars through diet alone or through both diet and insulin. With the aid of frequent blood sugar and urine tests, normal blood sugar levels can be maintained. Diet alone may be satisfactory for those who had mild diabetes before pregnancy or those with pregnancy diabetes. However, diet control alone has some drawbacks. Current medical thinking stresses that in pregnancy a fairly large number of calories is necessary to assure adequate nutrition of the infant. An average of 1700–2500 calories per day (from foods relatively high in calcium, protein, and carbohydrate) is recommended. The diet cannot be greatly restricted in an attempt to control the blood sugar, as it might be in the nonpregnant woman. Even the overweight woman who might otherwise go on a restricted diet must postpone such a diet until after pregnancy to avoid the potential hazards to the baby caused by undernutrition. A weight gain of 25-30 pounds during the course of pregnancy is now considered healthiest for the mother and baby.

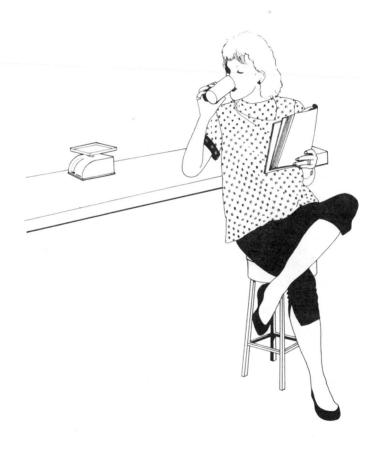

It is important that the woman understand all aspects of any diet and that she measure her food intake rather than estimate it, since estimated totals can be off by as many as 500 calories. Several visits with a diet counselor may be necessary in order to arrive at the proper diet. If 1700-2500 calories result in elevated blood sugar, then insulin will be needed. In those cases where a woman is introduced to insulin for the first time, it is appropriate for her to be hospitalized for complete instructions concerning insulin use.

The insulin-dependent woman will need the same type of diet as that prescribed for the diabetic woman whose diabetes can be controlled with diet alone. If blood sugars become elevated, then more insulin will be needed.

To monitor the effect of diet and insulin in the control of diabetes, several procedures have been developed. Although urine tests for sugar are often useful, it should be noted that in pregnancy there is a lowered renal threshold for sugar, so that blood sugar may be near normal at the same time that sugar appears in the urine. In cases of low renal threshold or incompatible results from urine and blood sugar testing, urine sugars are not reliable indicators for guiding insulin therapy. Therefore, blood sugars must be used instead.

While urine sugar tests are not especially helpful in monitoring insulin therapy, testing for urine ketones (acetone) *is* useful. Ketonuria can result from undereating (called "starvation ketosis") or from lack of insulin and poor diabetes control. Either condition is potentially harmful, and an appropriate change in therapy is indicated: either more food or more insulin (the latter if the patient is following the appropriate diet and is not overeating).

"Fasting" blood sugar and "after eating" (postprandial) blood sugar tests should be done anywhere from two to ten times per week, depending on the degree of control. If control is not good, more frequent blood sugar determinations may be necessary. Blood sugars should be kept between 60 and 120 mg%. If we assume that the mother is on the right diet, elevations above these levels may be an indication that more insulin is needed. Blood sugar determination can be obtained at the doctor's office, or possibly through the use of his lab. For more frequent blood sugars, the physician might be able to arrange for a machine (the *Accu-Chek bG* or *Glucometer*) to be used at home by the patient to test her own blood sugar, or the patient may be able to use *Chemstrip bG* as discussed in the chapter on home blood sugar monitoring. Any change in the therapy of a pregnant woman should be made under the supervision of the physician (medical or obstetric) taking primary responsibility for control of the diabetes.

It is important to monitor the general health of the pregnant woman as well as her blood sugar and urine acetone. This will mean fairly frequent visits to the doctor to measure blood pressure, to examine the eyes for retinopathy, and to check for other problems such as bladder infections. Any of these problems could be present without obvious symptoms, and routine examination can lead to early detection of any complications. If any problems are present, they should be treated at once.

The previous discussion has dealt primarily with keeping the mother in good health. Another important issue is determining the best time for the delivery of the baby. In the past, before diabetes could be controlled, there was a moderate chance that the baby would not survive a full-term pregnancy. Because of this, it was common to deliver the baby by Caesarean section early in the 33rd to 37th week. Sometimes this was too early and the baby was not mature or strong enough to resist disease. One frequent consequence of such an early delivery was respiratory distress (hyaline membrane disease) in the newborn.

Today, however, with the much improved methods of monitoring fetal progress, pregnancies can be prolonged in almost all cases until the baby is strong enough for delivery. These methods include measuring the fetus's heart rate in response to contractions of the uterus, measuring estrogen levels of the woman (which are usually very high in pregnancy), and using amniocentesis to measure the levels of lecithin and sphingomyelin (fats produced by the fetal lungs) in the fluid inside the uterus. The latter helps determine whether the fetal lungs will be mature enough to accept the job of breathing at birth.

These tests are usually done from the 32nd to 34th week on, at weekly or twice-weekly intervals, depending on how well the pregnancy is proceeding. Using their results, the physician will choose the best time and method of delivery.

By using the monitoring techniques that are currently available and by availing herself of proper medical care, the woman with diabetes can expect to give birth to a healthy baby. It does require her dedication, as implied by the foregoing discussion, and in many instances, some financial burden. But the reward of a healthy newborn makes any personal or financial commitment tremendously worthwhile.

The Menses

The *menses*, commonly called the "period," refers to vaginal bleeding that generally occurs in the woman every 28 to 36 days. In some women, the interval can be less than 28 days or more than 36 days and still be normal. This bleeding results from the sloughing off of the cells that line the uterus. These cells are affected by the female hormones, estrogen and progesterone, which are produced by the ovaries.

When fertilization does not occur, estrogen and progesterone become very low in concentration and cease to stimulate or nourish the cells lining the uterus. Bleeding results over the next 3 to 5 days until the estrogen concentration again starts to increase during the next menstrual cycle. Associated with the menses and related hormonal changes are several symptoms, including swelling of hands and feet, cramps, nausea, and irritability.

The *menarche*, or the age when the menses first begins, usually occurs around 12 to 14 years of age. When a woman has diabetes, the menarche may be somewhat delayed. This is particularly true when the diabetes has been poorly controlled because of insufficient insulin, overeating, or poor nutrition. This results in disturbance of hormonal balance and in impaired physical development. Once the female diabetic properly adjusts her insulin dose and adopts a more nutritionally balanced diet, the menarche should occur. If the menarche does not then occur, other medical possibilities should be explored to explain the condition. Sometimes it is normal for the menarche to start as late as 16 years of age, particularly if this is a family trait.

Poorly controlled diabetes can also affect the regularity of the cycle. It is uncertain whether mental stress, hormonal imbalance, poor nutrition, or other factors associated with poor control cause menstrual irregularity. In any case, good diabetic control usually means a more regular cycle.

Just as diabetes can affect the menses, the menses and associated hormonal changes may possibly affect diabetes. Diabetic women can easily manage and anticipate these effects with a little knowledge.

As the levels of estrogen and progesterone increase just prior to the menses, there is some resistance to the effectiveness of insulin which can cause elevated blood sugar. For the insulin-dependent woman, this may mean a slight adjustment in insulin (higher dose) or, as most women prefer, reduced food intake to counteract this tendency toward higher blood sugar. For the non-insulin-dependent woman, reduced food intake is also appropriate just prior to menses. Then, when the menses occurs, hormonal estrogen and progesterone production decreases and blood sugar levels tend to decrease, especially if nausea is present. For those using insulin, a smaller dose during the menses may help prevent this tendency.

The *menopause*, commonly referred to as the "change of life," is the point at which the menses stops, usually sometime after the age of 40. At menopause, there *are* great changes taking place. Ovulation ceases and there is marked reduction in estrogen and progesterone production by the ovaries. Accompanying these changes are a number of unpleasant symptoms including depression, headache, hot flashes, and, as the woman gets older, a tendency towards brittleness of bones and resulting fractures. These symptoms occur in varying degrees with different women, and some women barely experience any of them at all.

"Hot flashes" can be one of the more disturbing and potentially embarrassing symptoms of menopause. The term refers to the sudden onset of the sensation of heat waves passing through the body accompanied by excessive perspiration, weakness, and headache. They can occur less than once a day to more than ten times per day. For the diabetic woman, they can be even more exasperating as they may be confused with hypoglycemia reactions which cause similar symptoms. This confusion can greatly complicate proper diabetes control. For instance, if a woman mistakes her "hot flashes" for hypoglycemia, she would take extra sugar or food which may elevate her blood sugar level way above normal. Conversely, if she mistakes her hypoglycemic symptoms for "hot flashes," she may fail to take sugar, and her low blood sugar reaction will become even more severe. Fortunately, there are ways to avoid confusion. By testing urine with a sensitive urine test, or even better, by testing her own blood sugar with one of the self blood sugar methods that are now available, a woman should be able to tell whether her symptoms are due to hypoglycemia or menopause.

Depression also occurs in varying degrees during and after menopause. A full discussion of depression is beyond the scope of this book, but it is probably partially related to reduced estrogen concentration that occurs during menopause. For the diabetic woman, mental stress, overeating or undereating (often associated with depression), and use of any antidepressive medication can affect blood sugar metabolism and proper diabetic control.

Brittleness of bones that can occur in varying degrees during or after menopause can lead to weakness and fractures in some women. Since diabetes itself can lead to bone brittleness, menopause in the diabetic woman often compounds the problem. If weakness and fracture complicate the diabetes, exercise may have to be restricted.

There is some evidence that brittle bones may be prevented by a diet high in calcium (at least 800 mg per day) and adequate in vitamin D (400 IU). If a patient's diet does not allow for one quart of milk per day (which contains the above supply of calcium and vitamin D) or sufficient amounts of other foods high in these nutrients, an ample amount of calcium can be easily and cheaply obtained from two Tums per day. A vitamin D supplement should be added, however.

Given the above discussion on menopause, is there anything that can be done to alleviate these unpleasant symptoms? Since the symptoms seem to be a manifestation of reduced estrogen production by the ovaries, supplemental intake of estrogens should be considered. It has been shown that estrogen can definitely relieve some or all of the symptoms associated with menopause. However, there is controversy about the use of estrogen since some medical studies indicate that estrogen supplementation may be associated with a slight increase in incidence of cancer of the uterus. The use of estrogen is thus a complicated issue and women with particularly severe menopausal symptoms should consult their doctor.

XIX
Diabetes and the Man: The Problem of Impotence

I MPOTENCE refers to the inability of a man to obtain adequate erection of the penis during sexual intimacy. As discussed earlier in the chapter on warning signs of diabetes, impotence can indicate the presence of diabetes. For many men with impotence, there are underlying psychological factors involved. However, in a recent study (reported in the *Journal of American Medical Association* vol. 244, p. 2430), a group of 63 men with normal sexual function was compared with a group of 58 impotent men, and it was found that 12% of the impotent men had glucose intolerance, whereas there were no cases of glucose intolerance in the group of men with normal sexual function. This tends to suggest that before psychological problems are implicated as the culprit, an impotent man should first make sure he doesn't have diabetes. As discussed below, treatment of diabetes may cure impotence.

It has been estimated in various studies that impotence occurs in somewhere between 10 to over 50% of men with diabetes. Although psychological causes may certainly contribute to impotence in the diabetic man, underlying complications related to the diabetes can often be the more clinically significant factors. There is no doubt in my mind (I'm not sure all authorities would agree) that the fatigue, loss of energy, and possible weight loss associated with prolonged periods of uncontrolled diabetes can most definitely sap a man of his libido or desire for sex. In addition, poor control of diabetes may lead to infections of the penis and prostate gland, which could also contribute to impotence. I have seen many cases where improved diabetic control has cured these forms of impotence.

Before discussing the more chronic forms of impotence, it is important to know that there is another form of impotence that may occur in the diabetic which may not be related to the diabetes itself. I am referring to drug-induced impotence. There are many drugs that can cause impotence, particularly blood pressure medication, certain antidepressants, and some of the muscle relaxants. All of these drugs exert their desired effect (i.e., blood pressure regulation, antidepressive effect, or muscle relaxation) by influencing either hormonal or nervous system responses. Unfortunately, by influencing these responses, they can cause impotence as a side effect, since obtaining an erection is also under hormonal and nervous system control.

Therefore, if it is suspected that one of these drugs is causing impotence, it may be wise to vary the dose and type of drug so that the drug may continue to have its desired effect, if needed, without producing impotence as a disturbing side effect.

As the diabetic man gets older, there can be other reasons for impotence. Since an erection occurs by engorgement of the penis by blood, impaired blood flow caused by disease of the blood vessels (arteriosclerosis) is a fairly common cause of impotence. Even more common is "diabetic neuropathy," a nerve disease which affects the arteries and veins that control blood flow to the penis. Arteriosclerosis and diabetic neuropathy generally occur in diabetics who have had poor control of their blood glucose levels over a period of several years. Laboratory testing or a doctor's examination can usually verify whether or not impaired blood flow or neuropathy is present. If it is proven that either of these disorders is the cause of impotence, there are procedures performed by a urologist or vascular surgeon that can give excellent results. In view of the intricacy of these procedures, however, it is important for each diabetic to discuss the details of his particular condition with his doctor.

There's Hope!

For any man who may have a problem with impotence and who wonders whether things will ever improve, all is not lost. Take encouragement from a man I've been treating who told me how he lost his sex drive for two to three years. He knew something was wrong because he found that as he lay in bed with his wife each night, he did not have to resort to reading religious literature, as he customarily had in the past, in order to avoid stimulation of his sexual desire. His wife did not seem to mind very much, thinking that five children was enough, but *he* began to wonder, and so he sought my opinion.

His medical history showed that he had developed diabetes over the years. However, he had not followed any special diet, and he had not paid much attention to how well his diabetes was being controlled. After listening to his story and evaluating his condition, I suggested that better control of his diabetes through proper diet and exercise might well bring back his potency. I am very happy to report that once he followed these recommendations, my patient had cause to resume his old habit of reading religious literature (even more so after the birth of their sixth child) as he lay with his wife each night.

XX
Complications

THIS is the one chapter of the book I wish I did not have to write. Complications unfortunately *do* occur with diabetes. With the discovery of insulin in 1921, doctors hoped that we had the "cure" for diabetes. Certainly, insulin prevented the rapid progression from sickness to death in the insulin-dependent diabetic, but we have found that even with insulin, diabetics still suffer many complications. The death of the great Brooklyn Dodger baseball player, Jackie Robinson, who was the first black athlete to break into Major League Baseball, was attributed to diabetes complications. Cases such as his remind us that all diabetics may be susceptible to complications, and that insulin as we know it today is not a "cure" for diabetes.

What are the complications and how do they develop? In general, the diabetic's blood vessels take the brunt of the problems associated with diabetes. By affecting the blood vessels, diabetes can cause complications with the eyes, kidneys, nervous system, heart, and legs. There are two different types of blood vessel disease: small vessel disease and large vessel disease. Small vessel disease involves the eyes, kidneys, and nervous system, whereas large vessel disease involves the legs and heart.

Eye Complications

Small vessel disease is most striking in the eye. In the retina of the eye, there are many veins and arteries which are visible by looking through the pupil with a physician's ophthalmoscope. When diabetes affects these vessels, the veins become enlarged and twisted, and the arteries become narrowed. *Microaneurysms* occur, which are dilatations in the smallest vessels that lie between the arteries and veins. Associated with aneurysms are small, dot-sized hemorrhages. Occasionally, white or yellow spots are also seen. These dots, called *exudates*, may represent dead eye tissue that occurs when the blood vessels that should be supplying the necessary nutrients are impaired by diabetes. These eye changes discussed so far are referred to as *benign retinopathy* because, for the most part, they do not lead to loss of vision.

However, as diabetes progresses, and particularly when the diabetes has been poorly controlled, there can be leakage of fluid from the blood vessels and accumulation of the fluid in the retina (called *retinal edema*) which can result in loss of vision. In my practice, I have seen this condition many times. In some cases, however, when I feared that a patient's vision would continue to get worse, I found drastic improvement after the patient started to take better care of himself, controlling blood sugars, and possibly abstaining from alcohol. I am convinced that good control of diabetes is critical in curbing the development of these complications.

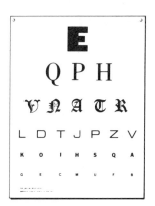

Another severe retinal disease is *proliferative retinopathy*, wherein the blood vessels of the retina proliferate (the reason is unknown), forming new blood vessels. These new blood vessels tend to bleed into the tissue called the *vitreous* of the eye and just behind it, causing impaired vision, retinal detachment, and even blindness. Up to 8% of diabetics may develop this type of severe retinopathy. Here too, many medical professionals believe that the more severe types of eye disease are rarely seen in patients who exercise and keep their diabetes under good control.

If proliferative retinopathy does develop, it is possible that partial loss of vision and blindness can be prevented with laser treatment. A major study, called the Diabetic Collaborative Study, was conducted in the 1970s by the National Eye Institute. In this study, patients with proliferative retinopathy had one of their eyes treated with a laser beam to prevent bleeding of the abnormal vessels, while the other eye was not treated. Results of the study indicated that the eye treated with laser therapy had far less vision loss than the eye not treated.

Because of the eye complications associated with diabetes, diabetics should have their eyes checked by a doctor experienced with diabetic retinopathy at least once a year. It is important for the diabetic to realize that serious changes can occur in the eye without any significant visual disturbance until blindness suddenly occurs. If the eyes are checked regularly, the problems can be identified before vision is impaired, laser treatment can be given, and blindness can be prevented.

Kidney Complications

Just as diabetes affects the eyes, it can also affect the kidney. If there are eye changes attributed to diabetes, there is a moderate chance that kidney changes are also present. The kidney contains a vast network of blood vessels, and in diabetics these blood vessels may become damaged and leak protein. This condition is signalled by protein in the urine, called *proteinuria*. In general, the diabetic usually has diabetes for more than 15 years before proteinuria occurs. Once it does occur, it is not uncommon to find other blood vessels in the kidney becoming sclerotic (hardened and narrowed). As these changes occur, hypertension may also result. Eventually, the kidneys may fail. Because of the serious implications of kidney disease, it is extremely important for the diabetic to have close medical attention.

Hypertension and kidney infections are particularly important warning signals of a diseased kidney. Treatment of these disorders may slow down the progression of the kidney disease. Current research also seems to indicate that good control of blood sugar helps retard kidney degeneration.

Nervous System Complications

Diabetic neuropathy is the general term used to describe pathology of the nerves. Nerve cells are very long cells emanating from the spinal cord or brain. Since the nerves connect to all the tissues of the body, diabetic neuropathy can affect the feet, joints, heart, muscles, stomach, intestines, and bladder.

When the feet are affected, loss of sensation usually occurs. This can start very subtly with numbness or "cold feet." As the neuropathy progresses, complete loss of pain sensation sometimes occurs. When this happens, the diabetic may be unaware that a cut, a blister, or even an infection is present until it has progressed to such a degree that it requires hospital care. This condition can be the precursor of gangrene, as discussed later in this chapter. Any patient with neuropathy of the feet should take all possible precautions, as outlined in the chapter on foot care.

When neuropathy involves the muscular system, it can result in weakness, clumsiness, muscle wasting, and even paralysis. Sometimes, the paralysis involves only one muscle, such as an eye muscle (possibly resulting in double vision). Frequently, however, this type of neuropathy is associated with inflammation of the nerves and therefore is called *neuritis*. The pain can be excruciating with this condition. The most severe cases of neuritis that I have seen occurred in diabetics whose diabetes was out of control for an extended period of time, and who had drunk excessive amounts of alcohol during this same time period. It is possible that a vitamin deficiency may also contribute to the neuropathy.

Paradoxically, it is not uncommon to see neuropathy temporarily exacerbated when attempts to control the diabetes are made; this sometimes occurs just after insulin is started so that the patient may even blame insulin for the condition. For the physician involved, this situation is particularly difficult because the patient can get discouraged if he doesn't see immediate improvement; and yet if attempts to control the diabetes are *not* made and sustained, the health of the patient is in serious jeopardy. In general, the condition stabilizes after four to six months of good control, and the neuritis pain becomes more tolerable. In the meantime, some medications (amitriptylene, phenytoin, fluphenazine) can be used with varying degrees of success.

Neuropathy can also affect the autonomic nervous system, which controls blood pressure responses, heart rate, heart contraction, bladder emptying, stomach and intestinal function, and sexual performance.

When blood pressure responses are affected by diabetic neuropathy, the blood pressure may fall drastically when the diabetic stands. This can result in decreased circulation to the brain and culminate in loss of consciousness.

When neuropathy affects the heart rate, there may not be an appropriate rate increase during stress or exercise, and blackouts can occur. Impairment of heart rate and heart contractions could cause heart failure (which means the heart does not pump blood properly), especially if the diabetic has a heart attack.

Neuropathy affecting the urinary bladder causes delay in emptying. Normally, it takes 200–300 milliliters (6–10 ounces) of urine in the bladder before a person feels the urge to void. With neuropathy of the bladder, however, this urge to void is lost, and the bladder may fill up with as much as one quart of urine and then not empty fully. This condition can lead to bladder infections.

Finally, when neuropathy affects the stomach and intestines, it can cause a variety of symptoms. Poor stomach emptying may result in distention of the stomach and periods of vomiting. A new drug, metoclopramide, has been partially successful in treating this problem. Constipation and diarrhea can also occur with neuropathy of the gastrointestinal tract and may require medical attention.

Complications of the Large Blood Vessels

Most of the above complications involving the eye, kidney, and nerves seem to have small blood vessel disease as their precursors. When diabetes affects the larger blood vessels, it may affect the legs, heart, and aorta. When the larger blood vessels to the legs are affected, the diabetic will have decreased blood flow due to *arteriosclerosis*, or hardening of the arteries. Arteriosclerosis may initially manifest itself by changes in the skin texture, loss of leg hair, and discoloration of the skin on the legs with blue mottling. As the arteriosclerosis progresses, cramping of the leg muscles occurs with walking or exercise. This condition is referred to as *intermittent claudication.*

Finally, *gangrene*, the most feared complication of diabetes, may occur. Gangrene refers to lack of blood supply to the affected part. Neuropathy and infection usually accompany gangrene and may ultimately lead to loss of a limb. My experience with gangrene is that in a large number of cases, neglect of wounds is at least partially responsible. I believe that most cases of amputation could have been prevented if there had been proper initial care of a simple wound.

Although the most feared complication is gangrene, the most life-threatening complication is heart disease. Diabetics have a much higher incidence of heart disease than the general population. In fact, if it weren't for heart disease, it is believed that non-insulin-dependent diabetics would live as long as nondiabetics. If a woman develops heart disease before menopause, there is a higher than average chance that she will have diabetes, whether or not it has manifested itself beforehand.

Why diabetics have greater incidence of heart disease is not fully established, but several areas of research seem to indicate that good control of diabetes can make a substantial difference. It has recently been found that if glycohemoglobin results are high, indicating that the control of diabetes is poor, there will often be an elevation of fats, cholesterol, and triglycerides in the blood. In addition, the HDL (high density lipoprotein) level in the blood, which serves as a protective factor against heart disease, is lower when diabetes control is poor.

Hypertension is another factor that may be responsible for the increased chance of heart disease in the diabetic. Diabetics have a higher incidence of hypertension, possibly because of kidney involvement, and this could contribute to the accelerated arteriosclerosis.

As long as I am discussing factors that influence the course of heart disease, I should address the issue of cigarette smoking.

First of all, in both diabetics and nondiabetics, cigarettes have an adverse effect on arteries, contributing to arteriosclerosis. There are three main arteries to the heart, called the *coronary arteries*, and arteriosclerosis affects these arteries, causing *coronary artery disease*. Cigarette smoking also affects other major arteries, such as those arteries in the brain and legs. There has even been evidence that cigarette smoking has adverse effects on the small blood vessels too. For instance, studies seem to indicate that diabetic smokers have a higher incidence of retinopathy than diabetic nonsmokers. Cigarette smoking *is* hazardous to one's health, and *especially* to the health of the diabetic.

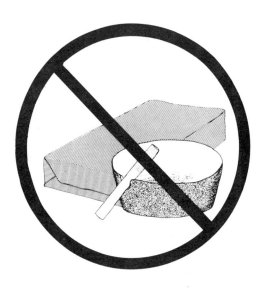

The typical symptom of heart disease is *angina pectoris*, which means pain in the chest. However, pain tends to vary in degree, location, and type. It may be a sharp pain, a tightness, a shortness of breath, or a sensation of gas in the chest similar to indigestion. Sometimes, it can be located in other areas besides the chest, such as in the jaw, arm, or elbow. It is frequently triggered by exercise or intense emotion.

Another indication of possible heart disease is *heart failure.* Symptoms of heart failure include fatigue, cough, and shortness of breath. I have seen heart failure not diagnosed many times, with the cough being dismissed as symptomatic of a cold or bronchitis. The cough and shortness of breath particularly occur at night, making it difficult to lie flat.

Finally, there are some diabetics who don't develop most of the symptoms associated with heart disease, particularly the symptoms of angina pectoris, despite the fact that they do indeed have heart disease. These patients have what is called *silent heart disease.* For some reason, possibly because of neuropathy which impairs the nerves that transmit pain, angina does not occur. It is very critical to be on the alert for this asymptomatic heart disease, particularly if exercise is recommended as a form of treatment, because if heart disease is present, the diabetic must exercise with caution. To diagnose this silent heart disease, a stress or exercise electrocardiogram should be performed. I recommend this test for any diabetic over the age of 40, especially if diabetes has been present for several years.

Find Out More!

Because this chapter only touches on the complications of diabetes, it would be worthwhile for the reader to learn much more about these complications by writing the American Diabetes Association for literature or by obtaining material from a local library or bookstore. Although I have heard many diabetics say they are not interested in hearing about the complications of diabetes, their failure to learn about them could prove dangerous, as in the case of Jackie Robinson. By knowing more about possible complications, the diabetic should fear them less, and will probably reach the conclusion that exercise, proper diet, and good diabetic control are the best ways to prevent the development of serious complications, at least until we discover new and better treatments for diabetes.

XXI
What To Do When Ill

KNOWING how to take care of yourself when you are ill should inspire confidence that diabetes can be controlled. With proper knowledge, you should have little fear of developing either diabetic coma with acidosis or coma from hypoglycemia.

Illness, even a minor one, often triggers elevation of blood sugar levels. For this reason, insulin-dependent diabetics often need more insulin, and those diabetics who normally control their disease without insulin may need doses of regular insulin during the course of their illness. Thus, many diabetics who don't normally take insulin might become familiar with the material in this chapter in case sickness necessitates insulin use.

Contrary to popular belief, "plenty of juices and fluids" is *not* good advice for a diabetic who is ill unless he knows exactly how these fluids are going to affect blood sugar levels. Consult your physician in this regard. Sugar and acetone tests should help you monitor the effects of your illness. If you are very sick, it is a good idea to have a friend or relative stay with you.

Sick Day Rules for Insulin-Dependent Diabetics

If you normally use insulin to control your diabetes, the most important rule during illness is *never omit your daily insulin dose*. Test your urine for sugar at least four times per day (before meals and at bedtime) and record the results. Depending on the seriousness of the illness and the results of the tests, more frequent testing may be required. You should also test your urine for acetone, especially if you are very ill. If you have negative sugar results but high acetone results, you may need to eat more carbohydrates. Call your physician, letting him know the results of your urine tests, the size of your usual insulin dose, and the extent of your fever.

If you are experiencing nausea and vomiting and are passing a lot of urine, take clear soups or salty broths every hour or so. These will help replace valuable salts and minerals. Note whether your tongue appears moist or dry. A dry tongue is a very important sign indicating that your body is losing more fluids than you are replacing.

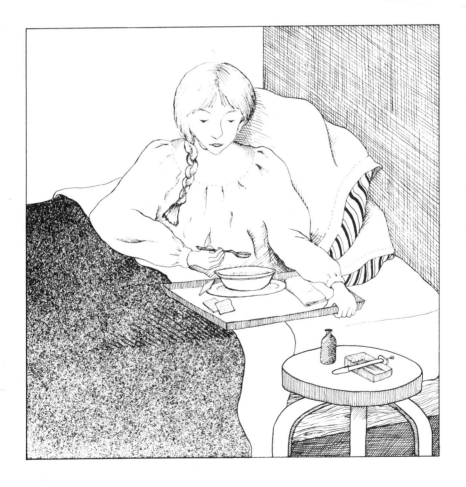

If you are able to eat your normal diet and the urine tests are consistently positive for sugar, you may need supplementary regular insulin. If you are eating less than usual, experiencing nausea and vomiting, and finding positive test results for sugar and acetone, you will definitely need extra regular insulin. The dose of regular insulin will vary according to many factors, especially the degree of the illness, the stage or type of diabetes, and the presence or absence of acetone. Follow the judgment of your physician. In general, however, the following rules apply:

- Take your usual dose of insulin in the habitual manner.
- Take additional regular insulin according to the following schedule if there are high levels of sugar and acetone in the urine.

Percent Urine Sugar	Doses of Additional Regular Insulin			
	7 AM	11:30 AM	5 PM	9 PM
If you take fewer than 16 Units a day, total (to include more than one kind of insulin) —				
1–5%	4 U reg	4 U reg	4 U reg	4 U reg
1/4–1%	2 U reg	2 U reg	2 U reg	2 U reg
Trace or Negative	—	—	—	—
If you take 16–40 Units a day, total —				
1–5%	6 U reg	6 U reg	6 U reg	6 U reg
1/4–1%	4 U reg	4 U reg	4 U reg	4 U reg
Trace or Negative	—	—	—	—
If you take more than 40 Units a day, total —				
1–5%	10 U reg	10 U reg	10 U reg	10 U reg
1/4–1%	6 U reg	6 U reg	6 U reg	6 U reg
Trace or Negative	—	—	—	—

If you are very sick and have a high acetone reading, more frequent urine testing and more insulin may be necessary. See discussion under ketoacidosis in the chapter entitled "Low and High Blood Sugar Reactions."

If you can't eat the foods in your regular diet, attempt to follow the diet outlined below, or the equivalent in other foods. This diet contains approximately 1200 calories. Although it may contain fewer calories than your usual diet, you probably don't have to worry about low blood sugar since your illness elevates the blood sugar as mentioned in the beginning of this chapter. That is also why it is important *not to skip* your insulin dose.

Sick Day Diet

Breakfast

    1/2 c. applesause
    1 poached egg on toast
    with butter *or* 1 oz.
    American cheese on toast
    Tea with lemon

10 AM

    1/2 c. cereal
    1/2 c. milk
    Tea

Lunch

    Broth (clear)
    2 oz. cottage cheese with
      1/2 c. canned dietetic fruit
    Saltines with butter
    Tea with lemon

3 PM

    3/4 c. orange juice
    Toast with butter

Dinner

    2 oz. slice chicken *or*
      small omelet
    Baked potato with butter
    Tomato juice
    Regular Jello

Bedtime

    1/2 c. apple juice *or*
      1/2 c. canned dietetic fruit
    Toast *or* 5 Saltines
    Tea with lemon

Cases of food poisoning or severe vomiting and diarrhea (gastroenteritis) are special instances when you may want to be cautious about taking your full dose of insulin. If the urine tests are negative for *sugar* and *acetone*, you may take one-half to three-quarters of the usual dose and take the rest when your appetite improves. If the tests are positive for sugar and acetone, the whole dose of insulin should probably be taken. If, in either of the above cases, vomiting or nausea continues for more than four hours, you may very well have more than just food poisoning or a virus, and you should contact your physician.

XXII
Alcohol's Effects

FOR many, alcohol can relieve tensions, complement a gourmet meal, and add to the conviviality of a social gathering, but in excess it can be deeply destructive. The diabetic will undoubtedly hear a wide range of attitudes about alcohol. Some doctors strictly forbid the slightest alcohol consumption for the diabetic, while others are more flexible and adjust their attitudes to the needs and condition of each particular diabetic patient.

Ten percent of the U.S. population suffers from excessive alcohol consumption, which can result in impairment of mental faculties, uncontrolled appetites, malnutrition, and personality changes. These consequences can eventually affect interpersonal relationships both at home and work, possibly leading to marital difficulties or the loss of a fine job.

The diabetic must be even more cautious with alcohol than the nondiabetic since alcohol can complicate diabetes, making proper control very difficult. Although gin, vodka, bourbon, scotch, and dry wine are not carbohydrates, proteins, or fats, they do contain calories which must be accounted for in the diabetic's diet. Despite the calories, alcohol does not contain the necessary minerals and vitamins needed by the body. It is very important not to "substitute" straight alcohol for a bread and fruit exchange (as had been previously recommended) because of its lack of nutrients and because such a substitution could greatly reduce blood sugar levels.

A full understanding of alcohol's effects is particularly critical for the insulin-dependent diabetic. A few drinks can reduce mental alertness, sometimes causing a diabetic to forget to eat. A delayed meal combined with the fact that alcohol can inhibit gluconeogenesis (the liver's formation of sugar from noncarbohydrates) can induce hypoglycemia and result in loss of consciousness. With alcohol on the diabetic's breath, this hypoglycemia may be mistaken for drunkenness, and this misconception could delay necessary treatment.

Drinking enough alcohol to cause nausea and vomiting or a "hangover" may greatly interfere with proper diabetic control since dehydration and reduced food intake can induce ketoacidosis. Furthermore, continual excessive alcohol intake can damage the nerves, causing pain in the legs and feet (neuritis), reduced reflexes, muscle weakness, or even paralysis. These symptoms mimic the symptoms of diabetic neuropathy. Some of the most serious cases of diabetic neuropathy that I have seen occurred in people with a long history of uncontrolled diabetes compounded by prolonged, heavy alcohol intake.

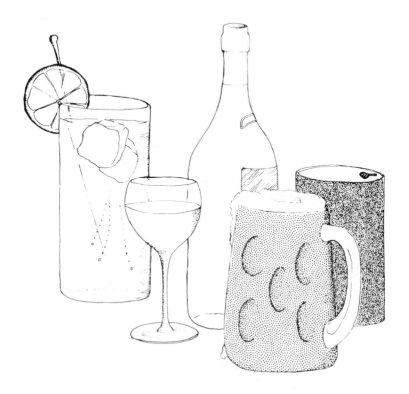

Another troublesome effect of alcohol is frequently seen in patients using the oral antidiabetic agent Diabinese. In some patients, alcohol combined with Diabinese causes flushing, nausea, and "hot flash" sensations. The mechanism behind these symptoms is not well understood. However, it is interesting to know that patients who suffer from these symptoms do not usually suffer some of the chronic complications that are seen in diabetes.

Calories in Alcoholic Beverages

I have seen so many patients who are completely ignorant of the calories in alcoholic beverages that it no longer surprises me. Patients state that they maintain their 1200 calorie diet perfectly and wonder why their diabetes is not controlled, not taking into consideration the caloric content of the alcohol they drink. I know of one patient in particular who kept to his 1200 calorie diet except for one thing — he drank a case of beer per day. When he eliminated beer from his diet, he lost weight, he could stop using the oral hypoglycemic agent prescribed to him, and his diabetes became controlled.

The caloric content of alcoholic beverages varies considerably. You may remember from the diet section of this book that carbohydrate has 4 calories per gram, protein has 4 calories per gram, and fat has 9 calories per gram. Alcohol is metabolized differently from carbohydrate, protein, or fat, and has approximately 7 calories per gram. In addition, there are varying amounts of carbohydrate and sometimes small amounts of protein in the different alcoholic beverages.

To simplify things, the American Diabetes Association (ADA) has recently published an alcohol exchange list reprinted on the following page.

This list does not include the sweet dessert wines nor the liqueurs (most of which have more than 30% sugar and are high in alcohol content as well) which should be avoided by most diabetics. In general, most of the dry white wines include *Chablis, Chenin Blanc, Pinot Noir,* and *Zinfandel.* Dry red wines include the burgundies. If there is *any* taste of sweetness, the wine should be consumed in less than 3 ounce quantities and should possibly be substituted for a fruit exchange, which brings me to the issue of mixed drinks.

Type of Alcohol	Ounces	Calories	Carbo-hydrate (g)	Exchanges
Rum, Whiskey, Gin, Vodka				
42 proof	1 ½	50	—	1 Fat
80 proof	1 ½	97	—	2 Fats
100 proof	1 ½	124	—	3 Fats
Beer	12	170	16	1 Bread, 2 Fats
Diet Beer or Light Beer	12	96	—	2 Fats
Wine				
Dry Table Wine	4	90	0–3	2 Fats
Dry Sherry	2	75	0–2	1 ½ Fats

It is not uncommon for people to mix a little juice with an alcoholic beverage in order to mask the bitter taste of alcohol. One such common drink is the *Screwdriver*, a blend of orange juice and vodka. The problem with this is twofold: first, people drink it as if it were plain orange juice, and second, the ease with which it is drunk may cause a double jeopardy — as the blood sugar is rapidly climbing, so is the blood alcohol content. However, if such beverages can be kept to a minimum, it may be reasonable to substitute an exchange or two in the diet depending on what is added to the alcohol in the beverage. A Screwdriver would be equivalent to one or more fruit exchanges, depending on the amount of orange juice. Beer might be substituted for one to two bread exchanges. Again, I caution you, however: just because your diet may allow 9 bread exchanges, you should not substitute 6 or 7 beers — the nutritional content is simply not the same!

I conclude, therefore, by saying that for those people who can enjoy an occasional drink, and not more than 2 light drinks on any day, it is likely that this minimal amount of alcohol will not have much effect on the diabetes. For those so inclined (providing they have the approval of their physicians), alcohol may be considered a cherished commodity, available to enliven the social and amicable spirits. To them: "SKOAL!" To the nondrinkers: "SKOAL!" as well.

Occasions When the Doctor Takes a Drink

Although I am acutely aware of the adverse effects of extreme alcohol consumption on the diabetic and nondiabetic alike, I do occasionally consume a beverage of high spirits. It is not unknown for me to celebrate a hard fought tennis victory with a beer to replenish the fluid deficiency from heavy exercise. I certainly will lift a glass of champagne to bring in the New Year or to offer a toast at a wedding celebration. Even a glass of dry, low-calorie wine can be seen passing my lips as I relax at home with my family in the evening.

XXIII
Foot Care

M ANY diabetics develop foot complications during the course of their disease. These complications include dry, brittle toenails; pain, tingling, or numbness of the toes and feet; sores on the toes and the soles of the feet; foot inflammations and infections; and night cramps in the legs. The most dreaded complication, gangrene, should be avoidable with special attention to general foot hygiene. The two main foot complaints in diabetics are neuropathy and poor circulation.

Neuropathy

As discussed earlier, neuropathy is best described as a loss or lessening of sensation. For example, if you were to step on a sharp object such as a tack and not experience pain, you may very well have diabetic neuropathy. There are varying degrees of loss of feeling. You may be aware of excruciating pain (as in gout or severe injury) but not of minor injuries such as stubbing your toe. You may not feel pain at the time but later notice a cut or bruise. The exact cause of diabetic neuropathy is not completely understood, but there seems to be some connection between prolonged periods of excessively high blood sugar levels and the severity of diabetic neuropathy.

Poor Circulation

Poor circulation, most common in people who have had diabetes for a long period of time, also contributes to foot problems. Circulation usually deteriorates with age, even in people who are not diabetic.

As discussed in the chapter on complications, diabetes can affect the small arterial vessels. Since those vessels in the feet are farthest from the heart, they become the prime targets for poor circulation. These blood vessels age more rapidly than normal and become clogged so that they are no longer able to transport enough blood to the feet. Since a sufficient blood supply is necessary for normal maintenance of body tissues, feet and legs are the first to become adversely affected when circulation is inadequate. An early indication of this condition is a cramp-like pain experienced when walking a moderate distance. Another early sign is poor healing of any abrasion or open cut. If a diabetic's feet look red when sitting, this is a later indication of poor circulation. It is important to pay attention to these signs and consult a doctor if any of them are present.

On a general note, if you are a diabetic, whether or not you use insulin, you should inform *all* of the doctors that treat you (including your podiatrist and dentist) that you have diabetes.

Daily Foot Care

To maintain proper foot care and avoid problems with your feet, it is necessary to perform a daily routine of general foot care, hygiene, and inspection.

Washing of Feet. You should wash your feet *daily* with warm water, *not* hot water. Check the water temperature with your hand. Hot water can burn your feet without your knowing it if you have neuropathy. When taking a foot bath, use only a mild, nonmedicated soap. If you prefer, a tub bath can suffice. After bathing, dry the feet *carefully*. Make sure to dry between the toes, without pulling the towel vigorously between them.

Feet Examination. Once your feet are clean and dry, examine them very closely in adequate light. If your eyesight is poor, have someone inspect your feet for you. Look for blisters, cuts, or scratches. Any break in the skin is a potential area of infection and should be treated at home with great care.

If you find a skin break or blister, apply a mild antiseptic such as isopropyl alcohol, Bactine, ST-37, Merthiolate, or Metaphen to the area. Then cover the area with a dry, sterile dressing and secure in place with nonallergenic tape such as "Micro Pore" or any other paper tape. Do not apply adhesive tape, moleskin, or other occlusive dressing directly over the infected area. Iodine preparations, carbolic acid, and creosol should *never* be used. Also do not use commercial preparations such as Lysol, Epsom Salts, or Boric Acid in foot soaks unless prescribed by your physician or podiatrist.

Never use hot water bottles or heating pads of any kind on your feet. At the first sign of pain, redness, or swelling, consult your physician or podiatrist.

Lubrication. After washing, drying, and inspecting the feet, apply a blended lubricating cream to your feet to prevent dryness and cracks in the skin. Eucerin, Nivea, Dermassage, and Alpha-Keri Lotion are good commercial preparations which restore moisture to the skin. Avoid the areas around the toenails and in between the toes. After lubrication, dust the feet with a light, nonmedicated powder (baby powder or corn starch), particularly between the toes.

Care of the Toenails. Cut nails short in the center and never below the juncture of the nail and the flesh at the corners. Never dig into the corners of the nails. File your toenails with a diamond-type file, and never file shorter than the end of the toe. If your toenails are thick, discolored, hard, and tend to split when being filed, have your podiatrist trim them for you.

Care of Corns and Calluses. Never cut corns or calluses since you do not have the proper tools or the skill and cannot achieve the proper position to do so. Chemical agents such as corn cures should also be avoided. Salicylic acid preparations destroy tissue without causing pain, and they are very dangerous.

Footwear

Never walk barefoot in or outside the home. Shoes offer more protection than slippers, but slippers with sturdy toes can be worn around the house to prevent injury from toe stubbing.

Since any object that creates pressure or a break in the skin may cause irritation or infection, you should inspect the insides of your shoes for foreign objects, nail points, and torn linings. Avoiding wet feet, wet shoes, or wet socks, especially in the winter months, should also help prevent foot infection.

Shoes and Slippers. It is very important to select your shoes carefully, making sure they fit properly, providing enough room for all the toes to be in their natural positions, and allowing for toe motion. New shoes should be broken in gradually to prevent blister formation. Avoid new shoes with pointed toes, since they prevent proper foot position. Open-toe or open-heel shoes should also be avoided, since they do not provide enough protection for your feet.

Socks. Make sure to wear machine-washable cotton or wool socks with your shoes and to change your socks *daily* to ensure cleanliness. Avoid mended socks as well as socks with seams or constricting tops. Circular garters or any other support garment that causes local constriction should not be worn since they prevent proper blood circulation.

Socks should always be large enough to allow considerable toe motion. If the toes overlap or are too close together, separate them with lamb's wool.

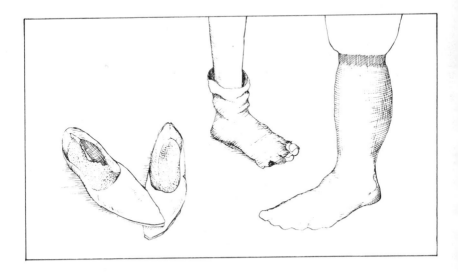

Final Tips

Three final tips related to general foot care are:

- *Do not smoke.* The nicotine in tobacco shrinks the blood vessels and slows down blood flow to the feet.
- *Avoid extreme temperatures.* Keep your feet at or above room temperature as much of the time as possible.
- *Exercise.* Walking improves circulation and is the best exercise for your feet.

XXIV
Diabetics Can Travel!

THE urge to travel is intrinsic to us all. We desire to move, to see, to go elsewhere and learn about faraway cultures different from our own. Having diabetes does not change this adventurous spirit and should not prevent exploration of the world around us.

Too often, however, diabetics give up their desire to travel and confine themselves to their homes, leaving only for necessities such as food and work. Their reasons for doing so may include ignorance of diet flexibility, fear of illness, or an assumption that travel always involves complex arrangements. The following points are some practical tips which should make traveling less threatening and more enjoyable.

Know your diet well. Consult your doctor or dietician if you have any questions. They should be able to help you choose the right foods, particularly if you are traveling to foreign countries where the basic foods are entirely different from those to which you are accustomed. Go to restaurants serving foods suitable to your diet. Weight Watchers, health food, vegetarian, and seafood restaurants should provide you with the essentials, but you must remember not to overdo a good thing. The typical American restaurant serves an overabundance of food, so when half-orders are not available, do not feel compelled to eat everything on the plate.

Remember to avoid fried foods, excess butter, and cream. Request a side order of dressing for your salad and a plain baked potato (without sour cream or butter) or other suitable bread substitutions. Although you don't want to eat excessively while on a trip, one or two meals per week in which you allow yourself to eat somewhat more heavily than normal should not cause much trouble. A little extra exercise on those days will help burn up the extra calories and keep the blood sugar down.

As for obtaining food while traveling by plane, most airlines are quite accommodating. If you are scheduling a long trip, an advance call to the airline will usually assure you of food that suits your diet. Even in cases when it is not possible to call in advance, most of the meals served aboard planes should not be much different from your usual diet. You should carry some food with you in case of unexpected delays, although in today's world it would be unusual not to have acceptable food readily available in such a situation.

For diabetics on insulin, a more than adequate insulin supply should be on hand in case part of it becomes lost. Insulin should be carried on your person, not in luggage where it can be affected by temperature changes. It need not be refrigerated and can be easily kept in your pocket. A small change in insulin dosage may be necessary during a day of heavy traveling or if the time change through which you are traveling exceeds four hours. It is wise to discuss this with your doctor before your trip.

Maintaining your diet when traveling by van is very easy since a van has plenty of storage room for food. Automobile travel may mean stopping more frequently, but again, you should have food in the car in case of traffic delays. Highway travel is convenient because of the many food facilities along the roadside. The big problem here is resisting the temptation of constantly available food. Remember, letting blood sugars run high by overeating may exhaust your energies and make your trip much less enjoyable.

When traveling by ship, it is important that you avoid seasickness, which can greatly aggravate your diabetes and cause other medical problems. Dramamine (dimenhydrinate) or a similar medication may prevent this problem.

"Traveler's diarrhea" is another disorder that may occur, especially in those traveling long distances from home. This condition is thought to be caused by bacteria in some foods, or simply by a drastic change in diet. Bottled rather than tap water should be used whenever possible to avoid possible reactions to various water purification methods. It may be worth having your doctor prescribe an antibiotic if you are traveling to locales where diarrhea is known to be a problem. You might also want to bring along medicines to control nausea and vomiting, such as trimethobenzamide (or Tigan), as well as medicines which alleviate diarrhea, such as loperamide (Imodium) or diphenoxylate (Lomotil).

Remember to bring on your trip some form of identification that states you are a diabetic. If you are traveling to a foreign country, it is also wise to contact the American Embassy in that country and get the names of English-speaking doctors.

In short, diabetes is no reason to inhibit travel. By knowing some basic information and taking some practical precautions, you can travel without substantial difficulties.

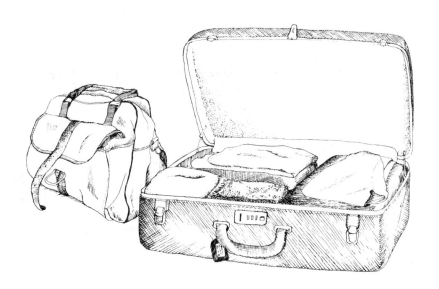

XXV
Diabetes After 50

ALTHOUGH more than ten percent of people in their sixties develop diabetes, this form of the disease fortunately tends to be mild and uncomplicated. Concentrated carbohydrates may need to be restricted in the diet, but there should be little change in lifestyle for the older diabetic. Recent information indicates that as one ages, there tends to be some glucose intolerance so that blood sugars may run somewhat higher. In other words, blood sugar levels that may be considered diabetic in a 20-year-old may be considered part of the normal aging process at age 70, as long as they are not excessive. To be more specific, most physicians would consider a 20-year-old patient a diabetic if he persistently had fasting blood sugars in the range of 130–140 mg% or above, but would avoid this diagnosis if the patient were nearing 70. Although I would not necessarily label a 70-year-old with those blood sugars as diabetic, I would probably offer him some advice. I would advise him against poor dietary habits and urge him to get what exercise he could. In addition, it would be important to have frequent medical checkups with particular attention to blood circulation, nervous system, and feet.

The onset of diabetes in the older person may coincide with a heart attack, gallbladder attack, or a number of other illnesses or infections. Blood sugars may climb to 500 mg% or more and insulin may be needed to get them back to normal. Once the illness is over, and an appropriate diet, high in fiber, is begun, blood sugars may improve and insulin can frequently be discontinued. These patients should then be treated in the same way as people with glucose intolerance.

Another common problem concerns the patient who has developed high blood sugars in the 200-350 mg% range but who is otherwise well, with no major health problems. It is hard to convince such a patient that he needs insulin. Of course, diet and exercise should be tried first, and an attempt to control blood sugars with the help of the oral agents may also be worthwhile. If the blood sugars respond within several weeks, the pills can then be stopped. If, however, none of these methods is effective in controlling the blood sugar levels, insulin therapy should be considered, depending on age and other relevant factors. The goal of insulin therapy in this case is to control fasting blood sugars relatively well, allowing some elevation of blood sugar after meals. This approach is less harmful than one which attempts perfect control and risks hypoglycemia.

Without question, insulin is helpful to many patients in their 60s, 70s, or 80s. There are many patients who have had such poor diabetic control despite proper diet, exercise, and maximum dosage of oral agents that they look like they are literally dying of cancer or starvation (and feel as if they are too). Insulin treatment for these patients frequently results in weight gain and increased strength and vigor.

For those patients who have had diabetes for several years, complications may be present. Since cases of older diabetics vary so widely, it is impossible to discuss them individually within the scope of this book. Hopefully, these diabetics are already well-informed about their particular type of disease and need no further explanation here.

XXVI
Research -
Quest for a Cure

E XERCISE, proper diet, appropriate insulin dosage, and general good health help reduce the risk of diabetes complications, but the possibility still remains that complications will occur. Research is needed to expand our understanding of diabetes and to enable us to treat the disease more effectively. Current research is very active, and there is good reason to believe that some of the questions about this complicated disease will soon be answered.

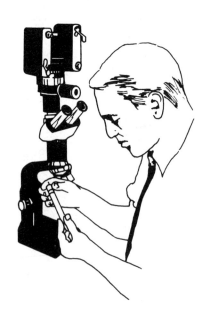

Viruses

In the forefront of diabetes research is the difficult task of discovering whether or not viruses are a possible cause of diabetes, especially the juvenile or insulin-dependent type. Mumps is the virus most commonly suspected as a possible cause of diabetes. Over the past 100 years, there have been many medical reports of patients who developed diabetes shortly after a mumps illness as well as reports on increased incidence of diabetes in the general population occurring after a mumps epidemic. In one medical journal, there was a report of a ten-month-old baby developing diabetes who did not have any of the usual characteristics of mumps but who did have two brothers who had had mumps shortly before the diagnosis of the baby's diabetes. The baby's doctors then performed blood tests to see whether or not the blood contained antibodies to mumps. Sure enough, antibodies were found.

This case is a good example of why it is so hard to implicate viruses. Viral diseases can be manifested by minimal symptoms, or so few typical ones, that the diagnosis is obscured. It is not uncommon for a patient diagnosed with sudden onset diabetes to have no recall of a previous illness that may in fact have triggered the diabetes.

In my own practice, I have often suspected that a viral factor is responsible for the onset of diabetes. In one particular family with no previous history of diabetes, two brothers and a sister all developed insulin-dependent diabetes; these siblings were all under the age of ten and they all had had mumps at various times before the onset of the diabetes. Although this information is suggestive, it is by no means conclusive when we consider that mumps affects over 70% of the population.

Besides mumps virus, numerous other viruses have been implicated as a cause for diabetes. These include hepatitis viruses, infectious mononucleosis virus, German measles virus, influenza virus (it was the influenza of 1968 that triggered my own diabetes; one day I was perfectly fine, the next day I had intense symptoms of diabetes along with symptoms of influenza), the common cold viruses, and more recently, a virus called Coxsackie B4 virus.

Other factors indicating the possible role of viruses include the following: 1) there seem to be seasonal peaks when diabetes occurs, corresponding to the times when these viruses are most active; 2) diabetes frequently occurs in patients who have no family history of the disease; 3) inflammatory cells are frequently found in the pancreas (where the beta cells are located) in patients with diabetes; and 4) antibodies to the beta cells are frequently found in insulin-dependent diabetes. Regarding this last point, people normally don't have antibodies to their own cells; thus, they shouldn't have antibodies to beta cells. However, if a virus attacks the beta cells or injures them, the beta cells could possibly act like foreign cells, causing the formation of beta cell antibodies, resulting in diabetes.

Researchers Dr. John Craighead in Vermont and Dr. Abner L. Notkins at the National Institute of Health have done extensive research on viruses and have demonstrated the development of diabetes by injecting mice with various viruses. When the pancreata of the mice were studied, there was microscopic evidence that the viruses affected the beta cells.

The most convincing case of a virus causing human diabetes occurred in 1978 when a young boy died with newly onset diabetes. At postmortem the doctors found damage to the beta cells. They then isolated from the pancreas a virus similar to the Coxsackie B4, grew the virus, and then injected it into mice. Some of the mice then developed diabetes. Although the case seems fairly conclusive, there is room for doubt since an estimated 40% of adults have antibodies to Coxsackie B4 and the proportion of diabetics is much smaller.

However, if it can be concluded that some forms of insulin-dependent diabetes are caused by a virus or viruses, then it is possible that a vaccine can be made which could make these types of diabetes as easily preventable as polio, smallpox, and other viral or infectious diseases.

Insulin

Considerable research is being done on insulin itself. As discussed earlier in the insulin chapter, we have come a long way in purifying insulin. Most of the insulin that is used today comes from the pancreata of cattle and swine. These insulins originally contained many impurities. Over the last ten years, most of the impurities have been eliminated so that insulins now used are over 99% true insulins.

Problems remain, however, with respect to the use of insulin from cattle and swine. Although these insulins are essentially purified, the insulin itself is slightly different in structure from human insulin. As you recall, insulin is a protein and is made up of approximately 51 amino acids. Pork insulin has one amino acid that is different from human insulin. Beef insulin has three amino acids that are different from human insulin. Thus, with the slight impurity and the slight variation of the presently available insulins, there is still the possibility of insulin allergy or insulin resistance (requiring large amounts of insulin to overcome the anti-insulin antibodies that the body produces).

Another problem is an economic one. It is estimated that it takes ten thousand pounds of swine and cattle pancreas to make one pound of insulin. With the current economic situation and the apparent increase of the incidence of diabetes, there is a distinct possibility that the supply of insulin from cattle and swine will run short. This shortage has already occurred in some countries.

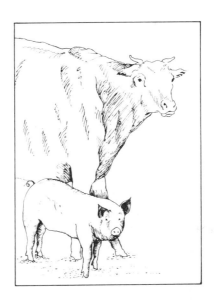

Some advances have been made in overcoming the allergy and insulin resistance associated with pork and beef insulins by the actual production of human insulin. There are several ways this can be done. Insulin can be made in the laboratory by linking amino acid constituents of human insulin together in the proper sequence. Apparently, this method has been used in several laboratories, but it is an impractical procedure because of the expense and the number of materials needed.

An alternative method of producing human insulin, introduced by the Novo Research Labs, replaces the amino acid in pork insulin (alanine) with the amino acid in human insulin (threonine). Novo Company is producing substantial yields of human insulin by this method and is now using it in several centers to determine its effectiveness.

Bacterially-Produced Human Insulin

Production of human insulin through the aid of bacteria may prove to be a more significant advancement. In late 1978, Genentech, a California-based company, developed a technique for producing human insulin through its genetic engineering research. In this technique, the human insulin gene or its components that control insulin production are synthesized in the laboratory. The synthesized gene components are then inserted into the DNA (genetic material) of the bacteria called *E. coli*. As the bacteria multiply, they generate the human insulin components which can then be extracted and combined.

The Eli Lilly Company, which is the largest manufacturer of insulin in the United States, is now using Genentech's techniques to produce human insulin. Some newly diagnosed diabetic patients have already benefited from its use on a research level. Pending FDA approval, it will eventually be available for clinical use.

There are probably other ways to manufacture *E. coli*-produced human insulin, but the scientific information is limited at present. The Eli Lilly Company, Novo Company, and Hoechst Company, all leaders in the diabetes field, are directing their attentions toward this goal. If the production of human insulin by these genetic engineering techniques can be perfected, we can expect a marked decrease in the incidence of insulin allergy and insulin resistance. Furthermore, there is potential for an unlimited source of insulin by these methods, which could make insulin much less expensive for the diabetic.

Insulin Pumps

Some diabetics, especially those who have had the disease for a long time, have "brittle diabetes," in which good control is virtually impossible because blood sugars fluctuate markedly with only minimal changes in food intake, insulin dose, or physical activity. Also, there is an increased tendency toward low blood sugar or high blood sugar coma.

Unable to achieve good control, patients may be more susceptible to some of the chronic complications. Doctors have been baffled by this condition, wondering whether patients were "cheating" on their diet, skipping meals or insulin doses, or whether their emotional state was having an adverse effect on control. However, even when these patients are hospitalized under controlled conditions, it is difficult to get perfect control despite good diet and frequent blood sugar monitoring.

Technological advances have introduced the possibility of managing this type of diabetes with the use of a portable infusion pump. There are several types of insulin pumps, all geared to deliver a steady amount of regular insulin every few minutes at a basal rate, so that over a 24-hour period approximately 15 to 30 units of regular insulin have been delivered. In addition, approximately 20 to 30 minutes before each major meal and heavy snacks, an additional amount of regular insulin (generally between 2 and 10 units) can be injected or "bolused."

Auto-Syringe, Inc. has been a pioneer in the development of insulin pumps and has recently introduced the *AS*6C*, which is an improved open-loop insulin delivery pump that allows independent control of both a constant basal rate and before-meal boluses. Essentially, the pump attempts to simulate normal, healthy pancreatic activity. Within seconds, basal rates are easily calibrated and can be quickly altered to meet insulin requirements. A digital display indicates the bolus delivery. This new pump is lighter, smaller, and more convenient than earlier pumps and has been a breakthrough in the research and development of insulin delivery systems.

Results of research studies on insulin pumps around the world have been striking. In some of these studies, patients with "brittle diabetes" have been able to maintain blood sugars that are close to normal for most of the day. The pumps have finally emerged from the research centers and are now being used in some patients. The following describes the use of the pump in a young man with diabetes that had been nearly impossible to control.

Man Helped By Pump

The man is presently in his mid-thirties. He has had diabetes since he was a teenager. When it was first diagnosed, he had difficulty controlling blood sugars and even had an episode of ketoacidosis. As he got older, he could prevent episodes of keto-acidosis and extremely high blood sugars, but blood sugars still bounced around excessively despite proper diet and regular exercise. In addition, he was prone to hypoglycemic episodes, some of which were quite severe. With this history, we brought him into the hospital hoping to achieve better control. His pre-hospital insulin dose was 34 NPH, 6 regular before breakfast and 6 NPH, 4 regular before supper. The following table shows this man's daily blood sugar levels and insulin dose (he was put on a diet of approximately 1800 calories). As the table indicates, we were hoping to get good control during this hospitalization with regular insulin before each main meal, along with intermediate-acting insulin NPH in the morning and before supper.

FIRST HOSPITALIZATION
WITHOUT INSULIN PUMP

Date	Blood Sugars (mg%)	Time	Insulin Dose (in units)	When Dose Was Given
Feb 13	357	Fasting or 7 AM	26 NPH 6 regular	before breakfast
	—	11 AM		
	255	3 PM	4 regular	before supper
Feb 14	125	7 AM	12 NPH 10 regular	before breakfast
	361	11 AM	4 regular	before lunch
	248	3 PM	6 regular	before supper
Feb 15	506	7 AM	12 NPH 10 regular	before breakfast
	550	11 AM	4 regular	before lunch
	356	3 PM	6 NPH 6 regular	before supper
Feb 16	386	7 AM	12 NPH 10 regular	before breakfast
	453	11 AM	6 regular	before lunch
	188	3 PM	4 NPH 4 regular	before supper
Feb 17	419	7 AM	12 NPH 12 regular	before breakfast
	513	11 AM	4 regular	before lunch
	322	3 PM	8 NPH 6 regular	before supper

FIRST HOSPITALIZATION
WITHOUT INSULIN PUMP (Continued)

Date	Blood Sugars (mg%)	Time	Insulin Dose (in units)	When Dose Was Given
Feb 18	564	7 AM	14 NPH 14 regular	before breakfast
	570	11 AM	8 regular	before lunch
	304	3 PM	8 NPH 6 regular	before supper
Feb 19	549	7 AM	20 NPH 10 regular	before breakfast
	543	11 AM	4 regular	before lunch
	213	3 PM	4 NPH 4 regular	before supper
		9 PM	4 NPH 4 regular	before bed
Feb 20	480	7 AM	32 NPH 6 regular	before breakfast
	500	11 AM	18 regular	before lunch
	96	3 PM	6 NPH	before supper

At this point, the patient had had enough (due to his lack of improvement) and discharged himself from the hospital.

Approximately six weeks later, we readmitted him in another effort to see if we could establish control with the help of an insulin pump. The following table shows the results.

SECOND HOSPITALIZATION
BEFORE PUMP STARTED

Date	Blood Sugars (mg%)	Time	Insulin Dose (in units)	When Dose Was Given
April 11		7 AM	36 NPH 4 regular	before breakfast
		11 AM		
	518	3 PM	6 NPH 4 regular	before supper
		9 PM		
April 12	123	7 AM	36 NPH 4 regular	before breakfast
	302	11 AM		
	179	3 PM	4 NPH 4 regular	before supper
		9 PM		
April 13	397	7 AM	20 NPH 10 regular	before breakfast
		11 AM	15 regular	before lunch
	402	3 PM	8 NPH 8 regular	before supper
	202	9 PM		
April 14	604	7 AM	20 NPH 10 regular	before breakfast
	590	11 AM	15 regular	before lunch
	307	3 PM	* * * PUMP STARTED * * *	

AFTER PUMP STARTED
(Basal Rate: 26 reg/24 hrs)

Date	Blood Sugars (mg%)	Time	Insulin Dose (in units)	When Dose Was Given
April 15	77	7 AM	9 regular	before breakfast
	160	11 AM	3 regular	before lunch
	156	3 PM	6 regular	before supper
	105	9 PM	3 regular	before night snack
April 16	177	7 AM	9 regular	before breakfast
	247	11 AM	3 regular	before lunch
	203	3 PM	6 regular	before supper
	177	9 PM	6 regular	before night snack
April 17	53	7 AM	9 regular	before breakfast
	141	11 AM	3 regular	before lunch
	117	3 PM	6 regular	before supper
	97	9 PM	6 regular	before night snack
April 18	64	7 AM	9 regular	before breakfast

This time the patient was tremendously pleased with his progress and the *doctor* discharged him from the hospital.

It should be noted that on the readmission date of 11 April his blood sugar was 518 mg%, and blood sugars remained well out of control until 15 April. The insulin pump was then started. The blood sugars that followed over the next four days were the best consecutive blood sugars that this man had had in at least as long as I've been following his condition. I saw him in a follow-up office visit several days later with a blood sugar of 84 mg%, the first normal blood sugar he had had in the office in ten consecutive office visits! In addition, his glycohemoglobin level, an index of diabetes control, fell from 10.9% (poor control) to 7.9%, which is in the normal range.

The use of the portable pumps is an exciting and encouraging new method of treatment. However, it should be emphasized that these pumps are not necessarily appropriate for everyone with diabetes; there are some potential drawbacks. As they appear now, the pumps are bulky and have to be worn on a belt, shoulder holster, or pouch of a garment. The site of injection is subcutaneous, as in an insulin injection, and the site has to be changed every 2 to 6 days. Patients feel "wired" to them as the insulin has to be given through a tubing from the pump. This may disrupt sexual activity for some people, although an understanding partner can do much to alleviate the diabetic's self-consciousness and frustration. In addition, pumps may interfere with some other forms of recreation, particularly swimming since some of the pumps are not waterproof. In such a case, the patient must detach the pump from the tubing while he swims and reattach it after the swim.

Another problem that patients should be aware of is that the pump may need "reprogramming" every so often. That is, there are times when more or less insulin may be needed. For instance, if you refer to the man just described, you can see he was programmed to get 26 units regular insulin basal rate, and 9 regular before breakfast, 3 regular before lunch, 6 regular before supper, and 6 regular before the night snack. If this man gets ill or overeats, he may need to take some extra insulin to get his blood sugars back to normal; if he overexercises, he may need slightly less insulin. Thus, at this stage in insulin pump development, it is obvious that these pumps are quite demanding.

But for those users who are satisfied with their improved diabetes control and the resulting sense of well-being, the inconvenience and demands of the pump seem a minimal trade-off.

Potential Improvements in the Insulin Pump

Further improvements on the insulin pump will focus on making them smaller and therefore easier to carry or wear. Progress is also being made in the design of an *implantable* insulin pump which would make this device even more convenient. However, implanted pumps would not be as accessible. Insulin would still have to be injected into the pumps, and they would have to have a remote-controlled program to adjust them when more or less insulin was needed, or to stop them in case of malfunction.

Another major ideal feature would be the development of a *glucose sensor.* Ideally, this sensor would constantly measure the blood sugar level and then relay a message to the insulin pump to automatically discharge more or less insulin in order to keep blood sugars in the normal range. The combined unit would in fact be an *artificial beta cell,* in that it would automatically adjust insulin in response to blood sugar levels.

Although this artificial beta cell sounds simple enough, it is quite a complicated thing to develop. Scientists have been working on the development of this glucose sensor for over ten years now, and millions of dollars have been spent without major success so far. Yet the prospects are brightening. Apparently, the greatest obstacle in the development of an implantable glucose sensor is making it compatible with human tissues. Just as the human body may reject a transplanted heart or kidney, it may also reject the glucose sensor. Researchers at centers such as the Joslin Clinic in Boston are hopeful that this rejection process can be overcome.

If this artificial beta cell becomes available, it would be superior to the portable insulin pump since it would allow for variations in food intake and automatically make adjustments in insulin dose to keep the blood sugar normal. Problems that remain to be solved include where in the body to place the insulin pump, how to get the insulin into the pump, and how to make sure the pump is working correctly.

Until more progress is made with insulin pumps and artificial beta cells, an alternative to the current electromechanical pump is the *Pen Pump* manufactured by Markwell Medical Institute. As the name suggests, it is the size of an ink pen. It consists of a disposable syringe and catheter as well as a special plunger that delivers precise doses of insulin. The modified syringe can contain 300 units of insulin. By rotating the plunger a full circle, 4 units of insulin can be administered. Waterproof and easy to use, the pump can be attached to underclothing, carried in a pocket, or hung from a chain around the neck.

Ideas vary as to what type of insulin combinations can be placed in the pump. My experience with it, after three months' use, is that regular insulin is most effective. I have been bolusing myself with regular insulin from the *Pen Pump* 20 to 30 minutes before each meal; and then, because regular insulin generally does not last more than 6 to 8 hours, I take an extra dose of lente insulin in the late evening to get some basal nighttime insulin. Theoretically, the same could be done with multiple injections of regular insulin, but the convenience of having a week's supply on a neck chain or in a pocket seems to be a major advantage. If the blood sugars are running high, it is easy to administer more insulin to bring them back down.

With the help of the *Pen Pump*, my fasting blood sugars have generally been below 120 mg% and my last glycohemoglobin was 6.2%. I have even been able to use the *Pen Pump* during heavy exercise. Worn on a chain, it has been no interference with my tennis game, much to the dismay of my opponents!

Pancreas or Beta Cell Transplantation

The above techniques offer encouraging possibilities in the effective treatment of diabetes through artificial devices. What about *live* techniques such as transplantation of healthy insulin-secreting cells into diabetic patients? Research into these possibilities has been going on for over fifteen years with the hope that this will lead to successful transplantation of either the whole pancreas or only the insulin-secreting beta cells themselves. It has already been demonstrated in experimental diabetic animals that diabetes can be reversed, at least temporarily, with either of these procedures. Even more encouraging is the fact that by reversing diabetes with these techniques, some of the diabetic complications that occur in these animals can be prevented, delayed, or even reversed with the use of transplants.

Theoretically, transplantation seems simple enough, but there are major problems. Transplantation of the whole pancreas is a risky operation. Infections, heart attacks, and the destruction of pancreatic tissue are serious life-threatening situations that would need to be addressed directly after surgery. Then there is the problem of pancreas rejection. The rejection process occurs because of the normal body's immune system which produces white blood cells and antibodies to the transplanted tissues. The only time that rejection would not occur is when the donated transplanted tissue is nearly identical to the recipient's tissue. In all other cases, large doses of powerful medication would be necessary to counteract this rejection phenomenon. These medicines have serious side effects, however, some of which make patients very prone to infection. Considering the problems involved, it is clear why transplantation of the pancreas has not been performed very often. In most cases of pancreas transplantation, the diabetes was complicated by life-threatening processes due to the many risks associated with the transplantation surgery. In some cases, there was considerable improvement in the control of the diabetes, but unfortunately, the extended life span of these patients was less than two years.

More inspiring in terms of transplantation is the research being done on the beta or islet cells themselves. It has been estimated that it only takes one ounce or less of beta cells to produce the desired insulin to control diabetes. Again, animal studies have been very encouraging, showing the reversibility of the diabetes. The operation is much simpler than transplanting the whole pancreas.

The problem remains, however, of how to procure enough of the beta or islet cells. The cells must come from the pancreas. In isolating the cells, much of the pancreas has to be destroyed as well. Once the cells are isolated, they must be preserved. Research is being done on how to obtain a greater quantity of cells.

When the beta cells are transplanted, they also can trigger the body's immune rejection process. As in the case of pancreatic transplantation patients, large doses of medication with potential dangerous side effects must be used to counteract the rejection process.

Another possible approach to overcoming beta cell transplantation rejection is finding a way to protect the beta cells from the immune system's antibodies and the attacking white blood cells. If the beta cells could be covered by a membrane which would prevent them from coming in contact with the antibodies or the attacking white cells, it would prolong the life of the beta cells. The membrane would have to be permeable so that oxygen, glucose, and other nutrients could pass through and nourish the beta cells. The other necessary function of this membrane would be to allow insulin to pass through it in response to rising blood sugar.

Advances in Non-Insulin-Dependent Diabetes

Much of this discussion centers on insulin-treated diabetes. But what about non-insulin-dependent diabetes which is by far the most common type? Here, too, much information has been accumulated over the last several years which may generate some answers. As discussed in earlier chapters, it has been found that 80% of non-insulin-treated or adult-onset diabetics actually have elevated blood insulin levels. Theoretically, the high blood insulin should keep blood sugar levels normal or even low, especially if the insulin levels are higher than normal. But for some reason, the body cells of the adult-onset diabetic *resist* the effect of insulin.

Normally, body cells have "receptors" which receive insulin so that it can keep blood glucose levels within a normal range. In the adult non-insulin-dependent diabetic, it is thought that these receptors do not function properly or that there are not enough of them. When this happens, diabetes develops despite high insulin levels. In addition, the high insulin levels may contribute to obesity, which further complicates the diabetes. Obesity, lack of exercise, and overeating may all contribute to the receptor defect. Medications that overcome this defect may be forthcoming.

Some insight into treatment of non-insulin-dependent diabetes may also be found in research work with glucagon. As indicated in earlier chapters, glucagon is a substance which, like insulin, is produced by the islet cells of the pancreas. However, it has the opposite effect from insulin: it raises blood sugar. Might the overproduction of glucagon be implicated in the development of diabetes? Most researchers think not, but efforts are being made to explore further this obvious possibility.

Glucagon has also been suspected as a cause of diabetic coma with ketoacidosis. There are some juvenile diabetics who are particularly prone to this type of coma. It has been shown that if glucagon blood levels can be suppressed, there will be less risk of ketoacidosis. Experimentation is presently being done with a substance called *somatostatin*, the third substance (in addition to glucagon and insulin) produced by the islet cells of the pancreas. Somatostatin has been shown to decrease glucagon levels and delay the onset of ketoacidosis in diabetic animals from which insulin is withheld. Somatostatin may have the same effect on humans. It remains to be proven, however, that somatostatin will have no serious side effects, and its effect must extend beyond just a few hours. At present, somatostatin must be given by injection, and this means the inconvenience of several injections per day.

Research on Diabetic Complications

What about some of the complications of diabetes? Have there been any advances in their treatment? With regard to eye complications, use of the laser beam has been successful in avoiding permanent loss of vision. However, it is essential to diagnose eye problems while they are in their earliest stages. It is also important to realize that severe retinopathy may be present without any visual impairment to alert the diabetic that loss of vision may soon occur. That's why it is of the utmost importance for diabetics to have frequent eye examinations by physicians who are familiar with diabetic retinopathy.

Impotence is another very frequent complication of diabetes. Recent studies indicate that impotence may be caused by damage to either nerves or blood vessels (arteriosclerosis) that supply the penis. It is not unusual for impotence to be the initial symptom leading to the diagnosis of diabetes, although current thinking is that diabetes is present for a considerable time before this symptom presents itself. It is possible that good control of the diabetes will relieve this symptom, but in cases where the nervous system or vascular system has been severely affected, it may be too late. (This is one more reason why early diagnosis of diabetes is important, so that treatment can be given as soon as possible.) Some success has been shown in recent work on blood vessels to improve the blood supply to the penis. Studies with male hormone therapy have shown no improvement in performance, although this type of therapy may stimulate sexual desire which is doubly frustrating under these conditions. Moderate success has been achieved through surgical penile implants which allow good performance during intercourse.

An additional complication that may plague the diabetic is neuritis, resulting from inflammation and disease of the nerves. It can cause extreme pain that can become unbearable, with associated sleepless nights, depression, and irritability. Numerous medicines have been used to control the pain, but in the last two years a combination of medicines (amitriptyline and fluphenazine) has proved to be somewhat effective. However, these medications themselves may have adverse side effects.

By now, it should be evident that while there is a tremendous amount still to be learned about diabetes, much has been accomplished. What we know about diabetes developed from work done hundreds of years ago by physicians and scientists who struggled to lay the groundwork for future research efforts. In medical research, steps can only be taken one at a time, and each step is very costly in terms of the money and time involved. It takes dedication and sacrifice on the part of the researchers, who give up the very considerable monetary rewards they could achieve in other fields. It is important that the public support the research efforts of these dedicated people. Both emotional and financial backing is needed so that researchers will not become frustrated at the slow rate of progress. Through the many diabetic associations, public support can sustain the morale of the researchers and the momentum of their efforts.

XXVI
Recommended Readings

B ELOW is a brief list of additional educational material that can provide the latest information about diabetes, nutrition, and exercise. This list is greatly abbreviated, and you should check the bookstore and library for the many other excellent books that can help you understand and manage your diabetes.

Diabetes Forecast — A bimonthly publication containing up-to-date diabetes information, including current theories about diabetes, dietary information, short biographies of famous people with diabetes or people who have lived many years with diabetes, as well as other helpful material. It can be obtained through the American Diabetes Association, 600 Fifth Avenue, New York, New York 10020.

The Pritikin Program for Diet and Exercise by Nathan Pritikin and Patrick M. McGrady, Jr., published in 1979 by Grosset & Dunlop, New York, New York. This book is a very controversial best-seller which has caused quite a stir in the medical community because of its drastic dietary recommendations. It proposes that 80% of the calories in one's daily diet should be in the form of high fiber carbohydrates, and less than 20% of the caloric intake should be in the form of protein and fat. Although there has been no definitive empirical proof that such a diet will indeed prolong the life span or prevent arteriosclerosis, this book makes some excellent nutritional points. It emphasizes the benefit of exercise in conjunction with proper diet, and there is no doubt that the Pritikin program can help control high blood pressure as well as diabetes.

The Sportsmedicine Book by Gabe Mirkin, M.D. and Marshall Hoffman, published in 1978 by Little, Brown & Company. Dr. Mirkin offers some provoking ideas about exercise and nutrition. Especially interesting is his discussion on the value of vitamins. He discusses programs for "peak" performance and suggests how injuries can be prevented and managed. This book may be very helpful to the sports-minded diabetic, even though it is not written specifically for the diabetic.

The Diabetic's Sports and Exercise Book by June Biermann and Barbara Toohey, published in 1977 by J.B. Lippincott. This is the first comprehensive book for the diabetic who exercises. It emphasizes the effectiveness of exercise in controlling diabetes and in lowering the insulin requirements for the insulin-dependent diabetic. The book is especially inspirational for the weight-conscious diabetic.

The Diabetic's Total Health Book by June Biermann and Barbara Toohey, published in 1980 by J.P. Tarcher, Inc., 9110 Sunset Blvd., Los Angeles, California 90069. Another very readable and thorough book by Biermann and Toohey.

The Calculating Cook by Jeanne Jones, published by 101 Productions, 79 Liberty Street, San Francisco, California 94110. This is an excellent book that shows how to create low-calorie gourmet meals. It also describes how foods can be made in quantity and then preserved, which is helpful to the individual who is hard-pressed for time.

Joslin Diabetes Manual edited by Leo J. Krall, 11th edition, published in 1978 by Lea & Febiger. This comprehensive work is written by physicians and other professionals of the Joslin Clinic where, for over 60 years, diabetes has been studied more intensely than in any other place in the world.

Diabetes: A Practical New Guide to Healthy Living by James W. Anderson, M.D., published in 1981 by Arco, 219 Park Ave. So., New York, New York 10003. Dr. James W. Anderson, a renowned expert in the diabetes field, outlines his highly successful ways of treating diabetes with special emphasis on how to incorporate high-fiber carbohydrate to help reduce the need for insulin in many patients as well as lower their cholesterol and blood fat levels.

INDEX

Accu-Chek bG, 39, 126
Acetest tablet, 33
Acetoacetate; *see* Ketone bodies
Acetone, in urine, 32-33, 69; *see also* Ketone bodies
Acidosis, 3; *see also* Ketoacidosis
Adult-onset diabetes; *see* Non-insulin-dependent diabetes
Age, diabetes onset and, 7, 160-161
Alcohol
  calories in, 149-150
  diabetes and consumption of, 10, 147-151
  Diabinese and, 149
  neuritis and consumption of, 137, 148
Alcohol exchange list, 150
Alpha cells, 65
American Diabetes Association
  diet management and, 87
  identification bracelets from, 72
American Dietetic Association, 87
Angina pectoris, 140
Antibodies, beta cell, 5
Antidepressants
  diabetes and, 130
  impotence and, 132
Arteriosclerosis
  as a complication of diabetes, 139, 140
  impotence and, 132, 178
  see also Blood vessels, complications in; Heart disease
Autoclix, 38
Autolet, 38

Bacteria, use in insulin production, 166-167

Banting, Frederick B., 4, 5
Beer; *see* Alcohol
Best, Charles H., 4, 5
Beta cells
  artificial, 174
  failure of, 5
  role of, 4
  transplantation of, 175-177
  tumors of, 19
  viruses and, 164
  see also Pancreas
Beta-hydroxybutyrate; *see* Ketone bodies
Birth; *see* Childbirth
Birth control pills, diabetes and, 10
Blood glucose
  abnormality in; *see* Glucose intolerance
  definition of, 2
  levels of, 3, 6
  see also Blood sugar levels
Blood pressure, high; *see* Hypertension
Blood pressure drugs, impotence and, 132
Blood sugar levels
  after-eating (postprandial), 23, 126
  differences between high and low, 71
  fasting, 20, 23
  illness and, 142, 145
  low; *see* Hypoglycemia
  menopause and, 130
  methods of home monitoring, 38-41; *see also* Blood sugar monitoring, home
  normal, 20, 23
  pregnancy and, 126
  unexplained high, 56
  see also Blood glucose

Blood sugar monitoring, home,
    34-41
  exercise and, 118
  glycemic index and, 112, 113,
    114
  insulin dose changes and,
    50-51
Blood vessels, complications in
    large, 138-141
Boils, 16
Bones, diabetes and brittle, 130
Bread exchanges, 88, 94-96
Breathing, deep; *see* Kussmaul
    breathing
Brittle diabetes
  a cure of, 43, 45
  insulin pumps and, 167-168
  treatment of, 167-173

Calluses, care of, 154
Calorie(s)
  amounts burned in activities,
    119
  definition of, 80
  in different types of alcohol, 150
Camps, diabetic, 116
Carbohydrates
  calories in, 80
  complex and simple, 1-4
  glycemic index and, 110, 112
  illness and consumption of, 143
  types and functions of, 81
Cellulose; *see* Carbohydrates
Chemical diabetes, 9
Chemstrip bG, 38-39, 41, 118, 126
Chemstrip K, 33
Chemstrip uG, 31
Childbirth, diabetes and, 127-128
Children, home blood sugar
    monitoring and, 36
Cholesterol, 82
  definition and function of, 83
  heart disease and, 139
  pectin and, 85

Cigarette smoking
  diabetes and, 139-140
  foot care and, 156
Circulation, poor, 152-153; *see
    also* Blood vessels
Claudication, intermittent, 139
Clinitest, 30-31, 32
Colitis, diet and, 87
Coma; *see* Diabetic coma
Complications
  diabetes-related, 134-141
  research on, 178-179
Contraceptives, oral; *see* Birth
    control pills
Corns, care of, 154
Craighead, John, 164
Cramps, leg, 153

Depression, diabetes and agents
    for, 130
Dextrometer, 39-40
Dextrostix, 39
Diabetes
  complications with, 134-141
  definition of, 1-4
  diagnosis of, 22-25
  exercise and control of, 118
  glycohemoglobin measurement
    and, 73-77
  impotence and, 131-133
  long-term control of, 73
  menstruation and, 128-130
  natural course of, 11-15
  pills for; *see* Diabetes pills
  predisposition toward, 10
  pregnancy and, 17, 123-128
  remission of, 12, 15
  research on, 162-179
  subtle signs of, 16-21
  symptoms of, 16, 22
  types of, 5-10
  viruses and, 5
  see also specific types
Diabetes Forecast, 180

Diabetes pills, 57-62
  interactions with other drugs, 61
  mode of action, 58-60
  recommended use of, 60-62
  UGDP study on, 57-58
  see also specific types
Diabetic Collaborative Study, 136
Diabetic coma, 10
  testing for potential, 27
  types of, 13
Diabetic diet; *see* Diet,
    diabetic
Diabetic ketoacidosis;
    see Ketoacidosis
Diabetic neuropathy; *see*
    Neuropathy, diabetic
Diabinese, 58-59, 149
Diastix, 31, 32
Diet, diabetic, 78-89
  danger of low-carbohydrate, 108
  definition of terms in, 80-85
  food exchange lists for, 90-103
  high-fiber, high-carbohydrate,
    low-fat, 87
  how to use exchange lists, 87-89
    104-106
  insulin and, 55
  insulin-dependent diabetes and,
    106
  pregnancy and, 124-126
  remission of diabetes with, 12
  sample meal for, 105
  see also Exchange lists; Weight
    loss
Drugs, diabetes and; *see*
    Diabetes pills; Insulin;
    specific drugs
Dymelor, 58-59

Eating, scheduling time of, 79;
    see also Diet, diabetic;
    Overeating

Emotional problems, diabetes
    and, 11; *see also*
    Psychological factors
Endocrine disorders, diabetes
    and, 10; *see also* Hormonal
    changes
Estrogen therapy, menopause
    and, 130
Exchange diet; *see* Diet, diabetic
Exchange lists; *see* Food
    exchange lists
Exercise, 115-122
  calories burned with types of,
    119
  diabetic coma with excess, 13
  foot care and, 156
  increase of insulin receptors
    with, 120
Exudates, 135
Eye complications, diabetes and,
    14, 134-136, 178; *see also*
    Vision complications
Eye diseases, exercise and, 121

Fat
  calories in, 80
  polyunsaturated, 82
  structure and function of, 82
  see also Cholesterol
Fat exchanges, 88, 100-101
Fatty acids, 82
Fiber, definition and benefits of
    dietary, 85, 87
Food, quick energy, 102
Food exchange chart, 103
Food exchange lists, 90-103
  alcohol, 150
  bread, 88, 94-96
  fat, 88, 100-101
  fruit, 88, 92-93
  glycemic index and, 112
  how to use, 104-106

meat, 88, 97-100
milk, 88, 90-91
vegetables, 88, 91-92
Food poisoning, insulin dose and, 145
Foot care, diabetes and, 152-156
Foot problems, diabetic
  neuropathy and, 137
Footwear, 154-155
Fructose, 2
  appetite and, 112
  glycemic index and, 110, 111, 113
Fruit exchange, 88, 92-93
Fungal infections, 16-17

Gangrene
  as complication of diabetes, 139
  avoidance of, 152
Genetics, diabetes and; *see*
  Heredity, diabetes and
Genetic engineering research, 166
Glucagon
  hypoglycemia and, 65, 122
  research on, 177
Glucometer, 40, 126
Gluconeogenesis, 67, 148
Glucose, 2, 3, 4, 7; *see also*
  Carbohydrates; Sugar;
  Glycemic index
Glucose intolerance, 9
  age and, 160-161
  impotence and, 131
  non-diabetes-related, 10
Glucose tolerance, impaired, 9
Glucose tolerance test, diabetes
  diagnosis and, 24; *see also*
  Steroid glucose tolerance test
Glucose sensors, 174
Glycemic index, 110-114
  sweets and, 112-114
Glycogen, 3

Glycohemoglobin test
  heart disease and, 139
  measurements and, 73-77
  as a therapeutic tool, 75-76
  values for, 74
Gram, definition of, 80

HDL; *see* High density
  lipoprotein
Heart disease
  cholesterol and, 83, 86
  diabetes and, 14, 21, 139
  exercise and, 120
  saturated fats and, 86
  silent, 141
  symptoms, 140-141
  see also Arteriosclerosis
Heart failure, 141
Hemoglobin, 73-74; *see also*
  Glycohemoglobin
Hemorrhage, eye, 135
Heredity, diabetes and, 7-8, 9
High blood sugar reactions; *see*
  Ketoacidosis
High density lipoprotein (HDL)
  definition of, 83
  effect of exercise on, 120
  heart disease and, 139
Home blood sugar monitoring;
  see Blood sugar monitoring,
  home
Hormonal changes
  diabetes onset with, 124
  hypoglycemia and, 21
  insulin blocks with, 124
  see also Menopause;
  Menstruation
Hormones; *see* Endocrine
  disorders; Estrogen therapy;
  Glucagon; Hormonal
  changes; Insulin; Male
  hormone therapy

Hypertension, diabetes and, 136-137, 139
Hypoglycemia, 63-66
  agents for; *see* Diabetes pills
  alcohol consumption and, 148
  confusion with "hot flashes," 129
  diabetes and, 18-19
  diabetic coma and, 13
  exercise and, 122
  non-diabetes-related, 19-20
  risk with meal skipping, 106
  symptoms of, 20
  treatment of, 65
  urine testing and, 27
Hypoglycemia-like disorders, 20-21
Hypoglycemia-like symptoms, home blood sugar monitoring and, 37

Identification, as a diabetic, 72, 154
Identification bracelets, 72
Illness
  diabetes and, 142-146
  home blood sugar monitoring and, 37
  insulin dose and, 142, 144-145
Impotence
  diabetes and, 21, 131-133, 178-179
  drug-induced, 132
Infections, diabetes and, 13, 16, 132
Insulin, 42-56
  availability and storage of, 47
  bacterially-produced human, 166-167
  brittle diabetes and, 43, 45
  cattle and swine, 165
  combining types of, 48-49
  diet and, 55

dose adjusting of, 49-55
  excess and coma, 13
  history of, 3-4, 42-43
  how to inject, 48
  injection sites for, 46
  receptor sites for, 6
  research on, 164-167
  tips on use of, 45-46
  types, onset and duration of, 44
  see also specific types
Insulin allergy, 165, 166
Insulin blocks, hormonal changes and, 124
Insulin-dependent diabetes, 5-6, 7
  causes of, 11-14, 163
  compared with non-insulin-dependent diabetes, 8
  diet for, 106
  exercise and, 117-118
  long-term complications with, 14
  pregnancy and, 126
  sick day rules and, 142-145
  see also Diabetes
Insulin dose
  adjusting of, 49-55
  illness and, 142, 144
Insulin pumps, 167-174
Insulin reactions, home blood sugar monitoring and, 36
Insulin receptors, 120, 177
Insulin resistance, 6, 42, 43, 69, 165, 166
  exercise and, 120
  menstrual cycle and, 129
  weight loss and, 120
Insulin treatment for ketoacidosis, 69-71

Joslin Clinic, 174
Joslin Diabetes Manual, 181
Juvenile diabetes; *see* Insulin-dependent diabetes

Ketoacidosis, 66-71
  diabetic coma and, 13
  illness and, 37
  symptoms and treatment for, 69-71
  urine testing and, 27
Ketone bodies, 68, 126; *see also* Acetone
Ketone testing, urine, 32-33
Ketonuria, 126
Ketostix, 33
Kidney complications, diabetes and, 136-137
Kidney disease, home blood sugar monitoring and, 36
Kidney threshold, low, 23; *see also* Renal threshold
Kussmaul breathing, acidosis and, 69

Lactose, 2
Latent chemical diabetes, 9
Legs
  cramps in, 153
  decreased flow to, 139
Libido loss; *see* Impotence
Lipoprotein, definition of, 83; *see also* High density lipoprotein
Low blood sugar; *see* Hypoglycemia
Low density lipoprotein (LDL) definition of, 83

Male hormone therapy, impotence and, 178
Meat exchanges, 88, 97-100
Medic Alert Foundation, 72
Menarche, 128
Menopause
  diabetes and, 129-130
  hypoglycemia and, 21
Menses; *see* Menstruation

Menstruation
  diabetes and, 128-130
  hypoglycemia and, 21
Microaneurysms, 134-135
Milk exchanges, 88, 90-91
Mumps virus, diabetes and, 163
Muscle problems, diabetic neuropathy and, 137

National Eye Institute, 136
National Institute of Health, 6, 164
Nausea, medicines to control, 159; *see also* Vomiting
Nervous system complications, diabetes and, 137-138; *see also* Neuritis; Neuropathy
Neuritis, 137-138, 148, 179
Neuropathy, diabetic, 137-138, 152
  alcohol consumption and, 148
  impotence and, 132
Non-insulin-dependent diabetes, 6, 7, 8
  course of, 14-15
  exercise and, 118, 120
  food exchange list use by, 104-105
  heart attacks and, 86
  remission of, 15
  research on, 177-178
  symptoms of, 10
Notkins, Abner L., 164
NPH insulin, 42, 44, 64
Nutrients, definition of, 81

Obesity, diabetes and, 18
Oral hypoglycemic agents; *see* Diabetes pills; *specific agents*
Orinase, 57, 58, 59
Overeaters Anonymous, 108

Overeating
  avoidance of, 78-79
  exacerbation of diabetes with, 12, 18
  weight loss and, 108
Overt diabetes, 9-10

Pancreas, 4
  diabetes and removal of, 10
  role of, 3
  transplantation of, 175-177
  see also Beta cells
Pauling, Linus, 83
Pectin, 85
Pen Pump, 174-175
Penis, surgical implants for, 178-179
Perfectionists, home blood sugar monitoring and, 37
Pneumonia, diabetic coma and, 13
Postprandial blood sugar; *see* Blood sugar levels, after-eating
Prediabetes, 9
Pregnancy
  blood sugar monitoring and, 36
  diabetes and, 17, 123-128
  urine testing and, 126
Pregnancy diabetes, 124
Pritikin diet, 112, 180
Proliferative retinopathy, 135-136
Prostate infections, diabetes and, 132
Proteins, definition and functions of, 82
Proteinuria, 136
Psychological factors, diabetes and, 5
Pump, portable infusion; *see* Insulin pumps; *Pen Pump*
PZI insulin, 42, 44, 45, 64

RDA; *see* Recommended daily allowance
Receptor sites, insulin, 6
Recommended daily allowance (RDA)
  definition of, 81
  of protein, 82
Regular insulin, 42, 44, 64
Remission, diabetic, 12, 15
Renal glycosuria, 23
Renal threshold
  definition and description of, 27-28
  home blood sugar monitoring and, 36
  pregnancy and, 126
Retinal edema, diabetes and, 135; *see also* Retinopathy
Retinopathy, 178
  benign, 135
  exercise and, 121
  proliferative, 135-136
Roth, Jesse, 6

Salicylic acid preparations, 154
Secondary diabetes, 10
Semilente insulin, effect of, 44, 64
"Shin spots," 17
Skin changes, diabetes and, 16-17
Smoking; *see* Cigarette smoking
Somatostatin, 178
Sports, diabetes and; *see* Exercise
Starch; *see* Carbohydrates
Steroid glucose tolerance test, 24-25
Sugar(s)
  definition and function of, 1-3
  diabetes and intake of, 5
  low blood; *see* Hypoglycemia
  simple, 2, 3
  see also Carbohydrates; Glucose; Glycogen

Sweeteners, noncaloric vs. caloric, 112-113
Syringes, 47

Tes-Tape, 30, 32, 77, 118
Tests; *see* Blood sugar monitoring; Glucose tolerance test; Urine testing
Thirst, diabetes and, 16, 22
Toenails, care of, 154
Tolinase, 58, 59
Transplants, beta cell, 175-177
Travel, the diabetic and, 157-159
Triglycerides, 82, 83
Type I diabetes, 5-6; *see also* Insulin-dependent diabetes
Type II diabetes, 6; *see also* Non-insulin-dependent diabetes

University Group Diabetes Program Study (UGDP), diabetes pills and, 57-58
Urine
diabetes and excess production of, 16
second voided specimens of, 29
Urine acetone, 69
Urine ketones, pregnancy and, 126; *see also* Ketone bodies
Urine sugar testing, 22-23, 29-32, 126
Urine testing, 26-33
acetone or ketone, 32-33
exercise and, 118
illness and, 142, 144
menopause and, 130
see also specific tests; Urine sugar testing

Vascular disease; *see* Heart disease
Vegetable exchanges, 88, 91-92
Viruses, diabetes and, 5, 163-164
Vision complications
diabetes and, 22, 134-136, 178
exercise and, 121
Vision loss, diabetes and, 14
Vitamin D, cholesterol and, 83
Vitamins
fat-soluble, 82
function, sources and RDA for, 83-85
Vomiting, insulin dose and, 145

Weight gain, pregnancy and, 125
Weight loss
diabetes and, 16
recommendations for, 107-109
Weight Watchers, 108
Wine; *see* Alcohol
Women
diabetes and, 123-130
vascular disease in diabetic, 21

**To order additional copies,
please see the reverse of this page.**

RMI Corporation

341 Broadway, Cambridge, MA 02139 (617) 661-8707

TO ORDER ADDITIONAL COPIES

If **A Diabetic Doctor Looks At Diabetes: His and Yours** is unavailable at your local bookstore, please fill in the information requested, separate this page along the perforated line, and mail it (along with your check, if applicable) to RMI Corporation, 341 Broadway, Cambridge, Massachusetts 02139.

Please send me _____ copies of **A Diabetic Doctor Looks At Diabetes: His and Yours** at a cost of $7.95 plus 5% (minimum $1.50) Shipping and Handling.

Enclosed is my check in the amount of $_____

Please charge to my Master Card
or Visa Account: Account # _____

Exp. _____ MC Interbank # _____

Authorized Signature _____

Ship to: _____
              Name

              _____
              Institution (if applicable)

              _____
              Street

              _____
              City   State   Zip